HAEMORRHOIDS

CURED BY
HOMOEOPATHIC MEDICINES

*"Unless causes are removed from beginning to end
the disease can reproduce itself."*

By

P. SIVARAMAN

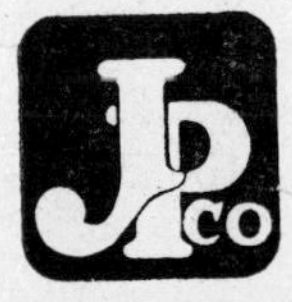

JAIN PUBLISHING CO.
New Delhi-110055

First Edition 1979

© JAIN PUBLISHING CO.

Price : **Rs. 6.50**

Published by : JAIN PUBLISHING CO.
2798, Rajguru Road,
New Delhi-110055.

Distributors : HARJEET & CO.
1920, Chuna Mandi, Paharganj,
Post Box No. 5752,
New Delhi-110055.

Printed at : New Light Printing Works
8145/7, Arakashan Road, Paharganj,
New Delhi-110055.

Preface

Specialization is an absurdity as far as medicines are concerned. Sickness in any organ means some disturbance in the economy of the sufferer, that means he becomes a PATIENT. Homoeopathy aims at curing the patient "rapidly, gently and permanently in the shortest, most reliable, and most harmless way on easily comprehensible principles," and not treating the DISEASE. Those who can only treat the sickness after naming it (diagnosis), those who believe that sicknesses are brought by germs and worms and viruses thereby aiming their medicine to destory these tiny poor creatures—as Don Quixote charging the supposed enemy—are not guided by medical science but by medical ignorance, and yet they exhort people to call them practitioners of MODERN MEDICINE. Their experiences are only with medicines or concentrated medicinal compounds administered on sufferers of sicknesses. These medicines are ever changing. Pharmaceutical firms are preparing and marketing medicines. The PATENT MEDICINES will crop up in the market for one or two years and a new set of medicines are marketed replacing the old ones. The so-called modern medical practitioners simply prescribe these medicines. There ends the NOBLE work of the learned physician. What action or reaction these concentrated medicinal compounds brings in the economy of the human being is not their concern. Ofcourse the primary action of the LIFE-SAVERS are suppression of the symptoms. The reaction lo ! and behold ! are entirely new diseases to them only to be named afresh and to be treated by still more concentrated compounds. This vicious circle goes on and on, and the poor patient is bounced from physician to physician and hospital to hospital. WHAT CAN THIS BE CALLED BUT MEDICAL IGNORANCE.

In the name of progress the world is rendered miserable to live in. The abnormalities caused by the effect of this so-called progress are many. Phosphates and sulphates, paramar and endrine are known poisons. The food we eat are cultivated using these and such other poisonous chemicals. Thus the food we eat, the water we drink, the air we breath in are all adulterated, contaminated and polluted. Can any sane man deny that these chemicals will not hamper the health of human being ?

I don't want to enter into a discussion and my aim is not that. Coming to our topic these allopathic brethren knows only of knife and some lotions. But from my experience I can testify that it can be cured by well selected internal homoeopathic medicines. Many homoeopathic brethren throughout the world will vouchsafe about the truth of this statement. And "truth never grows old."

The patient and the physician needs patience.

With these humble words, I submit this book to my homoeopathic brethren inviting suggestions and criticisms.

—THE AUTHOR

List of Medicines

Abbrn.	Name	Abbrn.	Name
Abrot.	Abrotanum.	Arn.	Arnica montana.
Acet-ac.	Acetic acid.	Ars.	Arsenicum album.
Acon.	Aconitum napellus.	Ars-i.	Arsenicum iodatum.
Aesc.	Aesculus hippocastanum.	Arum-t.	Arum triphyllum.
Agar.	Agaricus muscarius.	Aster.	Asterias tubens.
Agn.	Agnus castus.	Aur.	Aurum metallicum.
Alet.	Aletris farinosa	Aur-m.	Aurum muriaticum.
All-s.	Allium sativum.	Aur-m-n.	Aurum muriaticum natronatum.
Alos.	Aloe socotrina.		
Alumn.	Alumen.	Bapt.	Baptsia tinctoria.
Alum.	Alumina.	Bar-c.	Baryta carbonica.
Ambr.	Ambra grisea.	Bac.	Bacillinum.
Am-c.	Ammonium carbonicum.	Bell.	Belladonna.
		Berb.	Berberis vulgaris.
Am-m.	Ammonium muriaticum.	Bor.	Borax.
		Brom.	Bromium.
Anac.	Anacardium orientale.	Bry.	Bryonia alba.
Anag.	Anagallis arvensis.	Cact.	Cactus grandiflorus.
Anan.	Ananthereum muriaticum.	Calad.	Caladium seguinum.
		Calc.	Calcarea carbonica.
Ang.	Angustura vera.	Calc-f.	Calcarea fluorica.
Ant-c.	Antimonium crudum.	Calc-p.	Calcarea phosphorica.
Ant-t.	Antimonium tartaricum.	Calc-s.	Calcarea sulphurica.
Apis.	Apis mellifica.	Cann-s.	Cannabis sativa.
Apoc.	Apocynum cannabium.	Canth.	Cantharis.
Arg-n.	Argentum nitricum.	Caps.	Capsicum annum.

Abbrn.	*Name*
Carb-an.	Carbo animalis.
Carb-s.	Carboneum sulphuratum.
Carb-v.	Carbo vegetabilis.
Card-m.	Carduus marianus.
Carl.	Carlsbad.
Casc.	Cascarilla.
Caust.	Causticum.
Cham.	Chamomilla.
Chel.	Chelidonium majus.
Chim-u.	Chimaphila umbellata.
Chin.	China officianalis.
Chin-a.	Chininum arsenicosum.
Chin-s.	Chininum sulphuricum.
Chr-ac.	Chromicum acidum.
Cimx.	Cimex.
Cinnb.	Cinnabaris.
Clem.	Clematis erecta.
Cocc.	Cocculus indicus.
Colch.	Colchicum autumnale.
Coll.	Collinsonia canadensis.
Coloc.	Colocynthis.
Con.	Conium maculatum.
Cop.	Copaiva officianalis.
Croc.	Crocus sativus.
Crot-h.	Crotalus horridus.
Cycl.	Cyclamen europaeum.
Der.	Derris pinnata.
Dios.	Dioscorea villosa.
Elaps.	Elaps corallinus.
Elect.	Electricitas.

Abbrn.	*Name*
Erig.	Erigeron canadense.
Ery-a.	Eryngium acquaticum.
Euphr.	Euphrasia officianalis.
Ferr.	Ferrum metallicum.
Ferr-m.	Ferrum muriaticum.
Ferr-p.	Ferrum phosphoricum.
Fl-ac.	Fluoricum acidum.
Gamb.	Gambogia.
Gast.	Gastein.
Graph.	Graphites.
Grat.	Gratiola officianalis.
Ham.	Hamamelis virginica.
Hell.	Helleborus niger.
Helo.	Heloderma.
Hep.	Hepar sulphuris calcareum.
Hydr.	Hydrastis canadensis.
Hyos.	Hyoscyamus niger.
Hyper.	Hypericum perforatum.
Ign.	Ignatia amara.
Iod.	Iodium.
Ip.	Ipecacuanha.
Kali-bi.	Kali bichromicum.
Kali-br.	Kali bromatum.
Kali-c.	Kali carbonicum.
Kali-m.	Kali muriaticum.
Kali-p.	Kali phosphoricum.
Kali-s.	Kali sulphuricum.
Lach.	Lachesis.
Lact.	Lactuca virosa.
Lept.	Leptandra virginica.

| *Abbrn.* | *Name* | *Abbrn.* | *Name* |

Lil-t. Lilium tigrinum.
Lob. Lobelia inflata.
Lyc. Lycopodium clavatum.
Lycps. Lycopus virginicus.
Mag-m. Magnesia muriatica.
Manc. Mancinella.
Med. Medorrhinum.
Meli. Melilotus alba.
Meny. Meyanthes.
Merc. Mercurius.
Merc-bi. Mercurius biniodatus.
Mez. Mezereum.
Mill. Millefolium.
Murx. Murex.
Mur-ac. Muriaticum acidum.

Nat-m. Natrum muriaticum.
Nat-s. Natrum sulphuricum.
Nit-ac. Nitricum acidum.
Nux-m. Nux moschata.
Nux-v. Nux vomica.
Paeon. Paeonia officianalis.
Petr. Petroleum.
Ph-ac. Phosphoricum acidum.
Phos. Phosphorus.
Phys. Physostigma.
Phyt. Phytolacca decandra.

Pin-s. Pinus silvestris.
Plat. Platinum metallicum.
Plb. Plumbum metallicum.
Podo. Podophyllum.
Psor. Psorinum.
Puls. Pulsatilla nigricans.
Ran-s. Ranunculus sceleratus.
Rat. Ratania.
Rhus-t. Rhus toxicodendron.
Rumex. Rumex crispus.
Ruta. Ruta graveolens.
Sabin. Sabina.
Sang. Sanguinaria.
Sep. Sepia.
Sil. Silicea.

Stann. Stannum metallicum.
Staph. Staphisagria.
Sulph. Sulphur.
Sul-ac. Sulphuricum acidum.
Syph. Syphilinum.
Ther. Theridion.
Thuj. Thuja occidentalis.
Verat. Veratrum album.
Verb. Verbascum thapsus.
Zinc. Zincum metallicum.

PART I

MATERIA MEDICA

Rectum and Anus

The last twelve to fourteen centimetres of the alimentary canal is known as rectum. The last three centimetres is formed by the rectum. The rectum is dilated in the form of a flask (ampulla). Intestinal content, mostly waste (faeces), collects in the rectal ampulla.

Anus has two parts, one developed from the skin outside and the other from the intestine inside. It has got two layers of muscles, one longitudinal and the other circular, known as the external sphincter. At the upper end, it has the internal sphincter. Above the level of the internal sphincter is the rectum.

There will be a feeling of fullness when the faecel matter reaches the rectum. We can contract or relax the muscle ani to pass or retain the faecel matter at our will. Inside this muscle, there is a mucous membrane which is continued with the skin outside. Where it joins the skin it is known as anal-verge. The epithelium is columnal tissue. It is pink in the anus; this is known as the Venous-Plexus or Haemorrhoids. At the anal-verge, there is another plexus, called the external haemorrhoids.

In lower animals and the uncivilized, defecation is a reflex action that is set in motion as soon as the rectal ampulla becomes dilated. In the interests of decency and hygiene, the civilized are taught to inhibit this reflex and then to accomplish the act of defecation by a conscious effort at the proper time and in the proper place.

Whether through carelessness or lack of forethought, many of us permit large amounts of faeces to accumulate in the ampulla. The accumulated material tends to dry and cake (impaction of faeces), and the weight of impacted faeces causes the mucous membrane of the anus to protrude through the anal opening (prolapse). Unless the condition is rapidly corrected, the blood vessels of the prolapsed membrane become pinched off. At first they merely distend to form a haemorrhoid or pile that is still replaceable. But later, when the blood clots within their channel (thrombosed haemorrhoid), they cannot be replaced and are productive of extreme discomfort and pain. Sooner or later, the wall of the thrombosed pile tears or become storn during manipulation and the condition becomes one of a bleeding haemorrhoid.

The dilated veins form tumours of different sizes according to the amount of venous turgescence, from the size of a pea to that of a cherry or walnut, which sometimes encircle the entire anal opening like a bunch of grapes. When thus situated outside the anal margin they are called external, when within the anal margin internal haemorrhoids.

There are usually longer or shorter intervals between these spells of turgescence, during which the patient feels comparatively free from haemorrhoidal inconveniences. However repeated attacks of turgescence will gradually change either the mucous membrane or the submucous tissue, and produce catarrhal swelling of the mucous membrane, or hyperplasia of the connective tissue, or atrophy of these tissues under the influence of the pressure of the varices. The natural trugosities of the rectal mucous membrane become permanently thickened and inflamed, polypus growths are formed and associated with more or less pedunculated tumours, resulting finally in suppuration and consequent purulent discharges—white or slimy haemorrhoids.

The principal predisposing cause of the piles seems to be the position of the haemorrhoidal veins, as the lowest branches of the abdominal vessels, and in their want of valves to sustain the return column of blood in its course towards the vena porta. When a retardation or stagnation by some means or other in this backward moving column takes place, it is obvious that its whole weight must press downwards upon its lowest branches overfilling and dilating them. Such retardation of the refluent stream of blood may arise from different conditions.

1. From tumours within the abdominal cavity, which press upon the veins of the rectum; a gravid uterus; etc.

2. From the diseases of the liver, which obstructs the vena porta.

3. From diseases of the lungs, by which its capillaris become either obstructed or destroyed.

4. From diseases of the heart, by which the veins become overfilled with blood.

5. From a general relaxation of the abdominal veins, in consequence of using too much wine, coffee, tea or leading a sedantary life.

The fact, however that frequently all members of the same family suffer with this complaint, seems in favour of the assumption that piles are of a hereditary nature, probably

consisting of a congenital weakness or yirlding of the walls of
the haemorrhoidal veins.

Symptoms. As forerunners to their local appearance we
observe: fullness and pressure in the epigastrium, disturbed
digestion, bloating of the abdomen, costiveness, dull pain in
the small of the back, also in the head and nape of the neck,
hypochondriacal disposition, disinclination to work, and
especially to mental occupation, all symptoms which denote
a disturbed action in the abdominal organs. After a shorter
or longer duration of these sypmtoms, we find a gradual
development of the local symptoms at the anus—the beginning
of varicose veins, their gradual growth, their turgescence and
their collapse, alternating in longer or shorter intervals. Thus
the whole complaint is of a slow and tedious nature, changing
constantly from better to worse. The occasional spells of
bleeding are frequently attended with a feeling of relief,
though they do not better the morbid process itself in any
way; they become, in some cases habitual, assuming a regular
type of three to four week intervals. In such cases the
organism becomes so much accustomed to them, that
when they are suppressed in consequence of mental emotions,
or taking cold, or by external medical applications, etc.,
other disturbance set in, such as congestion of the head,
lungs, stomach, liver, kidneys, etc. which may result in
nosebleed, haemoptysis, bloody urine, apoplexy, etc.

In consequence of the stagnation of the return stream of
blood, which is caused by liver, heart or lung diseases, may
arise, also especially in older individuals, a varicose state of
the veins of the neck of the bladder, of the uterus or vagina,
causing haemorrhages from these organs, or slimy discharges,
painful micturition, etc.

Polypus of Rectum. The follicular or soft polypus occurs generally in childhood, very rarely in the adult, is attached to the mucus membrane by a narrow peduncle and usually protrudes in children after a stool, resembling a strawberry; it causes no pain but may produce bleeding sufficient to weaken the patient.

The fibrous or hard polypus is pear-shaped, with a peduncle more or less long and thick, protrudes if low down or attached to a long peduncle, causes some slimy discharge, but rarely bleeds, produces frequently the sensation of unrelief after stool, and its peduncle may be strangulated by the sphincter, which cause great pain.

Prolapsus Recti. The protusion of the hypertrophied mucus membrane, often observed in haemorrhoids, is not a true prolapsus. Thus, on the contrary, consists of a real falling down and out of all the coats of the rectum, is in fact an eversion of the gut, similar to intussusception, with this difference; that the falling of portion of the intestine becomes invaginated into that portion of the intestine which is just below it. The extent of the protrusion varies greatly, from three to fifteen centimetres, or even more. When not constricted by the sphincter it has the usual florid appearance; when strangulated it appears livid, purple and tumid from congestion. After long exposure the mucous membrane becomes thickened and granular and sometimes ulcerated.

Prolapsus recti is most frequently observed in children in consequence of protracted diarrhoea; less often it is found in adults, and then oftner in women than in men, in consequence of a weakened state of the sphincter, after childbearing, etc. The protrusion takes place usually during stool, sometimes after any movement, even when standing. The gut may remain constantly protruded, being fixed so as not to admit of replacement. In some cases the protruded portion has even sloughed off.

Fissura Ani. An anal fissure consists of an abrasion or ulcer usually at the posterior part of the lower circumference of the rectum, although it may occur in any other part of this portion of the anal mucous membrane, which here forms folds or pouches. When looked at without distending the rectum, the later edges only being presented to view, the ulcer appears like a fissure, but is in reality an abrasion or a superficial ulcer. On defacation its surface is irritated, extiting spasm of the sphincter muscle, and causing sharp cutting, burning and straining pains which last at times for two or three hours after stool. This trouble occurs usually in middle life and is more frequent in women than in men.

Fistula Recti. It is produced by the forming of an abscesses in the loose areolar tissue around the lower part of the rectum. After bursting outside near the anus its wall contract and become fistulous, forming a blind external fistula. If the suppurating process has at the same time opened a way through the rectal parietial into the bowel, it is a complete fistula. Blind internal fistulae, in which an opening leads into the bowel without an external orifice, are rarely met with, though it may happen that the original ulcerated opening in the rectum is so large as to allow the matter from the abscess in the areolar tissue to escape readily into the bowel without the necessity of burrowing its way through to the outside. Sometimes the sinuses are tortuous or pass in different directions and there may be more than one internal opening. At other times there is an external orifice on each side of the anus which leads to the back of the rectum and communicates with the gut at this part by a single orifice, so as to form a sort of horse-shoe fistula. In phthisical subjects a fistula may originate in consequence of tubercular ulceration and perforation of the bowel.

The forming of a fistula is always attended with pain, heat, redness and swelling before if breaks externally. Later, after the subsidence of inflammation and tenderness, it remains a constant annoyance by its discharging, more or less copiously, a thin purulent fluid when coming from a blind external fistula, or a brownish fluid from an admixture of feculent matter, when it issues from a complete fistula. At times the discharge becomes so thin and scanty that it appears as if the sinus were healing, when a fresh irritation again disappoints the sufferer.

Cancer of the Rectum. In the beginning of its development, when it causes a pressure upon, and a consecutive swelling of the haemorrhoidal veins, with occasional bloody discharges, and pain from the os sacrum down into the thighs it is most easily confounded with haemorrhoids. Later, however, the obstruction of the rectum becomes more apparent by the form of the discharged faeces, which appear pressed, flattened, angular, or pass off in small, hard nuts, like sheep-dung. Manual examination reveals now a knotted tumour, encircles the gut like a ring. In its still further advanced stage this tumour suppurates, and the bursting of blood vessels may occasion profuse haemorrhages. We sometimes observe in combination with it indurated inguinal glands.

Haemorrhoids

Abrotanum :

Protruding piles with burning from touch or passing stools.

Piles appeared and became worse as rheumatic pains abated, with frequent inclination to stool, hardly anything but blood being passed.

A suddenly checked diarrhoea followed by piles and acute rheumatism, with bleedings.

Oozing of blood and moisture from the navel.

Distension of abdomen.

Constant pain in stomach making the child irritable and ugly.

Flabbiness of skin hanging in folds.

Acetium acidum :

Profuse haemorrhoidal bleeding.

Haemorrhage from bowels after checked metorrhagia.

Malignant diseases of rectum.

Obstinate constipation, with great thirst and excess of pale urine.

Aconitum napellus :

Bleeding piles, with heat and sharp stiches ; inflamed ; stinging and pressure in anus ; blood bright.

Burning and heat in haemorrhoidal vessels.

Irritation of the haemorrhoidal vessels.

Abdomen feels full, with tensive, pressive colicky pains.

Bruised feeling in back and sacrum, inflammatory stage.

Sensation as of a discharge of warm fluid from the anus.

Aesculus hippocastanum :

Dryness, heat and constriction of the rectum.

Painful sensation of burning. Burning in rectum after stool.

Soreness, burning, itching and fullness in rectum, also in anus.

Pain in anus about an hour after stool, continuing for sometime.

Desire to strain at stool for a long time.

Large, hard, dry stools. Mucous membrane seems swollen and obstructs the passage.

Dry uncomfortable feeling in the rectum, as if it were filled with small sticks or splinters which were pricking the folds of mucous membrane.

Prolapsus ani after stool. Much pain after stool, with prolapse.

Haemorrhoids, with sharp shooting pains up the back.

Aching and lameness, or shooting in the back. Aching between shoulders.

Protruding engorged haemorrhoidal veins with backache, with absence of actual constipation. Weak feeling in sacroiliac joints as if leg would give way.

Constant dull backache, affecting sacrum and hips, much aggravated by walking or stooping.

Much pain but little bleeding ; if they bleed it gives relief.

Blind and bleeding haemorrhoids.

Abdominal plethora ; throbbing deep in abdomen, particularly in hypogastric region.

Fullness in various parts, as from an undue amount of blood.

Mucous membrane of mouth, throat, rectum, are swollen, burn, feel dry and raw.

All head symptoms accompanied by haemorrhoids, rectal or sacral symptoms.

Sore throat, chronic, with haemorrhoidal difficulty.

Pain like a knife sawing backwards and forwards through anus. Haemorrhoids like groundnuts, purple ; painful sensation of burning ; generally blind ; aching and lameness or shooting in the back. Haemorrhoids blind and painful ; rarely bleeding ; standing or walking. Stool hard, dry, and passed with difficulty. Sensation of rigid hardness before stool. Stools hard and black ; natural consistence and white. Backache after a difficult, large and hard stool. Prolapsus ani after stool. Several large piles which seem to block up the rectum, little or no bleeding, great suffering, constipation. Chronic diarrhoea, with characteristic backache or haemorrhoids. Piles develop and become particularly troublesome in climacteric years. Functional disturbances of the heart from haemorrhoidal complaints. The sacrum, back, neck, head, chest, heart and abdomen all seem in remarkable sympathy with the rectum and its vessels.

Characteristic backache. Constant backache affecting the sacrum and hips, very much aggravated by walking and stooping forward ; almost impossible to rise after sitting down. Back gives out when walking. Spine feels weak.

For persons with haemorrhoidal tendencies and who suffer with gastric, bilious or catarrhal troubles.

Worse during climateric, in winter, from standing.

After COLL. has improved piles, AESC. often cures. Useful after NUX and SULPH. has improved but failed to cure piles.

Agaricus muscarius :

Hard stools of a dark colour after a period of constipation. Tingling in anus.

Itching in anus, as from worms.

May have paralytic feeling of the rectum ; stool hard ; straining and sensation as if rectum would burst, even after stool.

Before stool, cutting and pinching in abdomen, can't wait ; distressing, bursting sensation.

During stool, colic and passing of flatus ; burning, soreness ; smarting and cutting in anus ; sweat ; pain in loins to legs, continuing after stool.

After stool, headache relieved ; biting in anus ; straining in rectum ; cutting pain in anus ; griping in hypogastrium ; distension in abdomen ; heaviness in abdomen and around navel ; pain in chest.

Agnus castus :

Difficulty of passing stools. When pressing at stool, discharge of prostrate fluid.

Sensation as of subcutaneous ulceration near the anus, only when walking.

Corrosive itching of the perineum.

Rhagades at the anus.

Deep fissures of the anus, often giving pain when walking.

Aletris farinosa :

Scanty diarrhoeic stool ; tenesums during and after stool, with feeling as if lower part of rectum closed.

Fearful pains in rectum and anus ; during movement terrible pains as if forcing a passage.

Inveterate constipation as from rectal atony.

Frequent ineffectual urging.

Stool ; loose, painful, offensive, frequent ; thin with hard lumps in it ; hard delayed, small scanty, difficult.

Haemorrhoids.

Allium sativum :

Normal stool immediately after a meal.

Stool delayed from morning until after dinner, great urging with stool, heat in rectum.

Constipation with almost constant dull pain in bowels.

Haemorrhoids.

Prolapsus ani.

Aloe socotrina :

Haemorrhoids ; large, prominent, tender, hot, like bunches of grapes with constant bearing down in rectum.

Burning in anus and rectum.

Haemorrhoids from a suppressed cutaneous eruption.

Haemorrhoids are mostly moist. Catarrh of rectum, which constantly secretes mucus and it escapes from anus at every attempt at defacation.

Constant bearing down sensation in rectum, with profuse emission of flatus before stool, followed by urgent diarrhoea especially in the early morning hours, hot and watery, with jelly-like mucus tinged with blood and followed by faintness aggravated after eating, in damp weather.

Want of confidence in sphincter ani, rectum feels full of fluids which feels heavy, as if it would fall out.

When urinating he has a feeling as though some liquid discharge from the bowels would take place at the same time.

Tendency to diarrhoea with the well-known uncertain feeling in the lower bowels *i.e.* flatus with faeces.

Much flatus with stool. When passing wind, feeling as if stool would escape with it.

Bowels feel as if scraped.

Itching, burning, pulsations, pain as from fissures at the anus ; preventing sleep. He is compelled to bore with the finger into the anus, so violent is the itching that the patient cannot let it alone ; it seems it will drive him to distraction.

Constipation, with heavy pressure in lower part of abdomen.

Before stool : rumbling ; violent sudden urging, heaviness in rectum.

During stool : tenesmus and much flatus.

After stool ; faintness ; cutting ; feeling as if more would come ; protruding piles.

Cold water ameliorates.

Alumen :

Haemorrhoids ulcerate : prolonged suffering after stool.

Asthmatic troubles with piles.

Dyspnoea during efforts to stool.

Severe pain in anus during stool and for some minutes after, better by bending forward and by pressure, worse lying on side.

Sharp pains in side of rectum.

Ulcers of rectum with ichorous, foetid or bloody discharge.

Violent itching around anus, especially evening and night.

Constipation.   There may be some urging to stool, without result or he may go several days without desire.   There is no ability to expel the stool.   He will strain a long time with no success, and finally after many days the stool is passed and is an agglomeration of hard balls large masses of little hard balls like marbles all fastened together.   There is a very strong feature in an ALUMEN consitiution "stool : less frequent dryer, and harder ; large black, hard or in small pieces like sheep's dung ; no relief afterwards." After stool there is a sensation as it the rectum were yet full.   This peculiar feature comes with the weakness or paresis of the rectum, *i.e.*, the rectum is not strong enough to expel all of its contents and hence the sensation of unfinished stool.   In the rectum there is ulceration with bleeding from the ulcers.   The haemorrhoids ulcerate and they are very painful, so that after every stool he has prolong suffering, a dull aching pain in the rectum.

A lumina :

Constipation of nursing children, from artificial food ; bottle-fed babies.

Inactivity of the rectum ; even the soft stool requires great straining.

No desire for and no ability to pass stool, until there is a large accumulation. Great straining, must grasp the seat of closet tightly.

The skin indurates and ulcerates and becomes clumsy and unhealthy and constipation is produced.

Stool hard and knotty like sheep's dung, covered with mucus ; with cutting in the anus followed by blood.

Must strain at stool in order to urinate.

Itching and burning at the anus ; fistula-ani.

Clots of blood escape from the anus.

Blood spurts out of the rectum during a stool ; followed by soreness all along the rectum ; sweat on perineum with tender-ness to touch ; moist varices sting and burn ; itching of anus with great sensitiveness.

Pressure and sense of excoriation in rectum after a small hard stool.

Excoriation in the anus after an evacuation, with contrac-tion of the rectum and constriction of the anus.

Haemorrhoids worse in evening, better after night's rest.

Blind piles protrude, become moist, with lancinating pain ; are hard and itch.

Fissures : He suffers greatly from constipation, he does much straining, the mucus membrane is thickened and swollen, and hence we have a fissure.

Before stool : Discharge of prostatic-juice, in rectum feeling of dryness and contraction ; chills.

After stool : Throbbing in spine ; stinging in anus.

Adapted to persons who suffer from chronic diseases ; "the Aconite of chronic diseases."

"When you see a remedy manufacturing and producing such a state upon the economy, growing that kind of mucous membrane that would favour fissures, you do not have to wait until you have cured a fissure with that remedy to find out if it will suit the case. You do not share to resort to the repertory to see what this remedy has done in fissure. From your general knowledge of the medicine you will see that it ought to cure the patient, as it produces such a condition of the mucous membrane and skin as would be naturally found in one who has a fissure. The skin indurates and becomes clumsy and unhealthy and constipation is produced, and so, after studying in that way, you are not surprised if it cures a fissure. You can also think over what other remedies you would expect to cure a fissure with. If you look into the nature of NITR-AC., CAUST., and GRAPH., you will see why they have had a wonderful record for curing fissure. That is the way to study your Materia Medica ; see what it does to the man himself, to his organs and tissues."

Ambra grisia :

Frequent ineffectual desire for stool, at this time presence of other persons becomes unbearable.

After the stool, pressure in the abdomen.

Large flow of blood with the stool, followed by pressure deep in hypogastrium, worse evening, lying down in warm place, on awaking, better from slow motion in open air and when lying or pressing upon the painful part.

Haemorrhoidal, excrescences in the anus.

Itching and tingling in the anus and in the rectum.

Increased urination, much more than the fluid taken.

Ammonium carbonicum :

After and during an evacuation, discharge of blood from the anus.

Haemorrhoids in the anus, sometimes bleeding, with smarting pains.

Haemorrhoidal tumours protruding before, during and after stool.

Protrusion of haemorrhoids from the rectum after stool, with long lasting pains, cannot walk ; protrude also independent of the stool.

Bleeding piles ; at every menstrual period bleeding from rectum.

Piles during menses, protrude, ameliorated lying down.

Haemorrhoids protrude during a stool, and recede when lying down.

Stools difficult, hard and knotty ; later, soft stools.
Costiveness on account of hardness of faeces.

Itching at anus and burning, preventing sleep must rise from bed on that account.

Before stool : Cutting pain in belly.

During stool : Straining and cutting pain in belly.

After stool : Scratching and burning in anus ; discharge of blood and prostratic juice, cutting pain in belly.

Ammonium muriaticum :

Hard crumbling stools, requiring great effort to expel them ; must use the abdominal muscles.

Hard stool covered with glairy mucus.
Green mucus stools alternate with constipation.
Constipation and piles with bleeding at stool.

Haemorrhoids sore and smarting, after suppressed leucor-rhoea.

Haemorrhoids surrounded by inflamed pustules, with itching and soreness.

Haemorrhoids : burning, stinging, smarting soreness.

Bleeding from rectum, with lancinating pain in perineum, especially evenings or when walking.

Much burning in rectum and anus during and for hours after stool.
Marked excoriation around the anus.
A heavy ring of warts around the anus with copious moisture.

Fig warts of the anus with the ulceration.

Before stool : Flatulency, colic.

During stool : Stinging, stitching, burning. and soreness in anus ; colic.

After stool : Pain in belly.

Anacardium orientale :

Bowels inactive.

Ineffectual desire ; rectum seems powerless, as if plugged up ; spasmodic contraction of sphincter ani ; even soft stool passes with difficulty.

Itching at anus.

Oozing of moisture from the rectum.
Painful haemorrhoids (both blind and bleeding) in the anus.
Fissures of the rectum.
Evacuation of blood with the stools.

A very characteristic sensation is a pressing or penetrating pain as from the PLUG, which may occur in any locality in connection with neuralgias and ear affections, piles, etc. and whenever present ANACARDIUM will probably be the remedy.

During stool : Pain in belly ; discharge of prostrate juice.

After stool : Abdominal pain ; gaping and eructation.

Anagallis aruvensis :

Itching in rectum.
Pressure in sacrum.
Piles.
Passes offensive flatus.

Anantherum muriaticum :

Stool mucous, bloody, brownish, yellow; whitish; choleriac ; offensive, with colic and burning in abdomen and rectum.

Obstinate constipation, stool hard, knotty, like sheep's dung.

Haemorrhoids and abscesses.
Itching at anus.

Angustura vera :

Pressive and contractive pain in the anus, with swelling of the haemorrhoids.

Burning in the anus while at stool.

Haemorrhoids protrude with hard knotty stool.

Antimonium crudum :

Difficult hard stools ; faeces too large. Constipation.

Hard lumps mixed with watery discharge.

Alternate constipation and diarrhoea.

Haemorrhoidal complaints due to constant over-indulgence.

Piles ; burn, prick, continuous discharge, stains yellow or sometimes ichour oozes out ; troublesome, in old gouty constitutions.

Constant oozing from the anus with or without piles.

Constant oozing of mucous, very disagreeable to the patient and emitting a sort of disgusting odour.

Mucuous piles, pricking and burning.

Haemorrhage from haemorrhoids. Flow of black blood.

Haemorrhoids are always sore and inflamed from a cold, wet day, from cold bathing and always worse if he is foolish enough to drink sour wine and take sour food.

Haemorrhoidal excresences, blind and running, with burning and tingling.

Burning itching and fissures in the anus. Burning furunculus in the perineum.

Expansive pressure in the rectum (during stool as if an ulcer had been torn open) and the anus.

During stool : Burning itching ; scraping and drawing in the anus ; stitching, scraping, soreness, and prolapse of rectum.

Antimonium tartaricum :

Desire for stool ineffectual, though the bowels seem full and pressing.

Constipation alternating with diarrhoea.

During the evacuation, palpitation of the heart.

Stitches and lancinations in the rectum.

Tenesmus during and after stool, frequent burning at the anus.

Apis mellifica :

Constipation, feeling in rectum as if it were stuffed full, with heat and throbbing ; feels as if something would break on straining.

Burning pain, excoriation of anus and constant tenesmus.

Prolapsus ani with haemorrhage from the bowels.

Small protruding varices, which sting, burn and smart intolerably.

Haemorrhoids with stinging pain after confinement.

"The stools are generally involuntary escaping continually from the wide open anus which does not close even after the stool is over. The patient complains of the anus feeling raw and sore. Haemorrhage from the bowels may also be present. The above symptoms may be complicated with haemorrhoids when the stinging, burning and the soreness already complained of assure a fiercer form."

Before stool : Straining.

During stool : Straining, pinching, nausea, vomiting, frontal headache, backache.

After stool : Exhaustion, approaching faintness.

Apocynum cannabium :

Bowels sluggish or diarrhoea, with sphincter ani so weak that faeces escape unhidden or while passing flatus.

All gone feeling in abdomen.

Haemorrhoids with a feeling as if a wedge were being hammered into the anus.

Argentum nitricum :

Constipation and dry faeces.

Tenia or ascarides with itching at anus.

Burning in one spot in a anterior wall of rectum.

Piles with burning or tenesmus ; bleeding.

Before stool : Abdominal pains.

During stool : Flatus, straining to vomit ; vomiting of slime, cramp of stomach ; drawing in abdomen ; difficult respiration.

After stool : Pain in stomach.

Arnica montana :

Constipation with ineffectual urging to go to stool.

Stools in the form of pap, of an acrid odour.

Flatus, smelling like rotten eggs.

Diarrhoea with tenesmus.

Frequent, scanty, small, mucus stools.

Stools of undigested matter.

Involuntary stools, chiefly during the night ; thin ; brown or white.

Purulent bloody stools.

Haemorrhoids. Pressure in the rectum. Tenesmus.

Prolapsus ani from overstraining and violent riding, worse from standing and from cold things.

Blind piles, with painful pressure in rectum, easily protruded from weakness of the parts.

Pain in anus as if it were bruised.

Before stool : Distension of abdomen.

During stool : Rumbling and pressure in abdomen ;—head-ache.

Arsenicum album :

Anus red and sore. Burning in anus.

Haemorrhoids ; with stitching pain when walking or sitting, not when at stool.

Haemorrhoids burn like fire, relieved by heat.

Painful spasmodic protrusion of rectum.

Haemorrhoids of drunkards.

Burning in rectum after stool, with weakness and trembling in all limbs.

Tenesmus with burning pain and pressure in rectum and anus.

Evacuations excoriate the anus.

Itching and eczematous eruption about the anus with burning.

Haemorrhoids are exceedingly painful as if burning needles plunged in.

Prolapsus of the rectum ; with much pain.

Itching, pain as from excoriation, and burning in the rectum and in the anus, as well as in the haemorrhoidal tumours, chiefly at night.

Shooting in the haemorrhoidal tumours.

Fissures of the rectum that bleed at every stool, with burning.

Fissures of the anus with impossibility of voiding urine.

Haemorrhoids bluish, swollen, inflamed, protruding and bunched, bleeding from least touch, with stitching, burning and soreness in rectum and anus, worse at night ; rectum is

spasmodically pushed out with great pain and remains protruded after haemorrhage from rectum ; irreducible strangulated haemorrhoids ; rhagades at different points with ichorous
discharge ; fissures with burning pains ; burning in epigastrium ;
restless and debility, worse at night, from cold, from ice-cream
and ice-water in hot weather ; better from warmth.

Before stool : Chilliness, anxiety, fainting, cutting in abdomen, vomiting, thirst.

During stool : Chilliness, nausea, vomiting, headache,
straining and burning in anus and rectum.

After stool : Cessation of acute abdominal pains ; distension,
straining about the navel ; burning in rectum ; oppression,
eructation ; weakness with trembling and faintness, with desire
to lie down ; palpitation, perspiration.

Arsenicum iodatum :

Very troublesome constipation.

Diarrhoea alternating with constipation.

Stool hard, knotty and light coloured.

External piles.

Itching of anus.

Burning in anus after stool.

Arum triphyllum :

Painful urging, with rumbling ; tenesmus towards evening.

Fissura ani, with retention of urine.

Burning at the anus.

Asteria rubens

Obstinate constipation, 12 to 15 days without stool, which was of hard round substances size of an olive.

Constipation, with ineffectual urging to stool.

Heat in the rectum : haemorrhoidal tumour ; piles.

Aurum metallicum :

Constipation or hard knotty stools.

Looseness and costiveness in alternation.

Piles with rectal catarrh, external piles bleed during stool.

Pain in small of back, as from fatigue.

Great nervous weakness.

Aggravated during menses with prolapsus uteri.

Aged people, pining youths, syphilitic subject, worse from mercury.

During stool : Pinching pain in abdomen ; burning in the rectum.

Aurum muriaticum :

Haemorrhoids, bleeding during stool.

Condylomata.

Anal and inter-crural excoriation.

Fistula.

Aurum muriaticum natronatum :

Clay like faeces.

Appearance of the haemorrhoid which protrude and is painful.

Baptisia tinctora :

In autumn or in hot weather, constipation ; severe with haemorrhoids : in afternoon stricture from piles.

Baryta carbonica :

Scanty, hard and lumpy stool, expelled with difficulty.
Frequent small stools, with great relief.
Constipation, with hard knotty stools ; haemorrhoids burning and soreness.
Moisture exuding from piles.
Burning in anus and rectum.
The anus is sore and humid.
Frequent passage of blood, with distended abdomen.

Itching, sensation of burning, excoriation and oozing at the anus.

Appearance of haemorrhoidal excrescences, with shooting pain.

Haemorrhoids protrude, not only with the stools, but also with urination.

Before stool : Colic.

During stool : Burning in anus and rectum.

After stool : Burning in anus, moisture exuding from piles ; eructation.

Bacillinum :

Severe haemorrhages from bowels, cough.

Obstinate constipation.

Passes much ill-smelling flatus.

Stitch-like pains through piles.

Belladonna :

Much straining, but passes scanty stool.

Mucous membrane of anus seems swollen as if pressed out.

Congestion of blood to head, red, hot face.

Piles so sensitive that the patient has to lie with the nates separated, or with a sensation as if the back would break.

Incarcerated varices from spasmodic constriction of the sphincter ani with great pain from the slightest touch.

Haemorrhoids that are violently painful, that are intensely red, that are greatly swollen and inflamed, a high grade of inflammation.

The haemorrhoids are painful and there is much burning.

Stinging pain in rectum ; back pains as if breaking.

Bleeding piles.

Before stool : Constriction in the rectum ;—some aching in upper part of abdomen ;—perspiration.

During stool : Shuddering ;—nausea and pressing pain in stomach.

After stool : Tenesmus.

Berberis vulgaris :

The patients become constipated, but the stool is white, or very light colour. Burning, stinging pain before, during and after stool. Enlargement of prostrate glands, which causes a constant pressure in the perinaeum. Pressure as if there were lump or as if something was pressing down. Tearing extending around the anus. Herpes around the anus.

Hard stool, like sheep's dung, passed only after much straining.

Violent burning pain in the anus, as if parts around it were sore, frequent and constant desire to stool.

Tearing, stitching, burning, crawling, or itching in and around anus.

Long continued sensation in rectum after stool, as if one had just been to stool, or had just recovered from a pain in anus.

Soreness in the anus, with burning ; pain when touched, and great sensitiveness when sitting.

Haemorrhoids, with itching and burning particularly after stool, which often is hard and covered with blood.

Fistula in ano with painful pressure in perinaeum, extending deep into pelvis (left side).

Constant pulsating stitches in sacrum.

Great soreness, and pain throughout back, from sacrum to shoulders, worse by any physical labour.

Acts forcibly on the venous system, producing pelvic engorgements and haemorrhoids.

BERBERIS produces both constipation (sheep's dung stools) and diarrhoea, and a number of symptoms about the anus.

Borax :

Itching, contraction, and shootings, in the anus and in the rectum.

Thickening of the mucous membrane of the rectum, with stricture, growing smaller and smaller until finally a long thin stool is passed, no larger than a pencil.

Bromium

Haemorrhoids, blind, painful, during and after stool, worse from application of cold or warm water ; better wetting with saliva (with black diarrhoeic) stools.

Haemorrhoids protrude from the rectum, burning, smarting day and night.

During the stool the rectum is painful from haemorrhoidal tumours.

We have running through the remedy enlarged veins. These are found in the rectum. Another symptom is that the stools in BROMIUM are generally black faecel stool.

Bryonia alba :

Chronic constipation, with severe headache.

Stool unsatisfactory, after much straining with rush of blood to head.

No desire; or urging with several attempts before result.

Stools hard, dark dry; as if burnt; too thick, too large.

Obstruction from induration of faeces.

Distended abdomen; rumbling and cutting, yet obstinate constipation.

After stool long-continued burning in rectum.

Hard, tough stool with protrusion of rectum.

Long lasting, burning in rectum after hard stool, or sharp burning pain in rectum with sharp stool.

Sensation of plug in anus.

Aching haemorrhoids.

Before stool : Colic ;—nausea.

During stool : Burning in anus ;—prolapse of rectum ;—motion like fermentation in abdomen ;—pain in stomach ;—vomiting, coldness and rigors; thirst ;—drowsiness.

After stool : Burning in rectum ;—heat ;—sleepiness.

Cactus grandiflorus :

Hard black stools.

Sensation of great weight in anus and urging to evacuate a great quantity, but nothing passes.

Constipation as from haemorrhoidal congestion.

Haemorrhoids swollen and painful.

Swollen varicies outside the anus, causing great pain.

Fluent haemorrhoids; copious haemorrhage from anus, which soon ceases.

Itching of anus; pricking in the anus as from sharp pains, ceasing from slight friction.

Fistula in ani with violent palpitation of heart.

CACTUS G. is a remedy for the cure of haemorrhoids; the relaxation of the great portal system, and the lower veins in rectum, the haemorrhoidal veins. The veins are in such state of relaxation that tumours will form, and bleed copiously. Bleeding haemorrhoids. Constriction of the anus. It has a troublesome constipation; constipation in connection with haemorrhoids.

Caladium seguinum :

Soft, scanty, pasty, clay-coloured stools, passed with difficulty.

Stool containing hard lumps.

Urging to stool on rising in the morning.

Burning in the anus after stool.

Stitches in rectum after stool.

After stool thin red blood passes.

Discharge of mucus from the rectum after stool.

Calcarea carbonica :

Constipation; stool at first hard, then pasty, then liquid.

Tendency to diarrhoea and acid stomach, and prolapsus recti; precussory of tuberculosis of lungs.

The constipation is generally complicated with haemorrhoidal affections and it is mostly mucous haemorrhoids.

Burning in the rectum and in the anus, with itching and tingling.

Burning eruption, in the form of a cluster, in the anus.

Cramps, tenesmus, and contraction of the rectum.

Cramps in the rectum the whole forenoon; a griping and stitching with great anxiety, was not able to sit, but obliged to walk about.

Excoriation at the anus, and between the buttocks, and the thighs.

Great irritability of anus, even a loose stool is painful.

Haemorrhoids which make even a loose stool painful, they are often painful when walking.

Intense aching and shooting in rectum, hours after stool.

Swelling, and frequent protrusion of haemorrhoidal excrescences especially during the evacuation with burning pains. Swollen haemorrhoids protrude and cause pain during stool.

Haemorrhoidal tumours appear, which pain both during motion and repose, and especially at stool, [and bleed freely. Frequent and copious bleeding piles.

Flow of blood from the anus during the evacuations also at other times.

Oozing and heaviness in lower portion of rectum.

Affections of the rectum, as fissures, which are very painful, bleeding after every stool, followed by extreme exhaustion.

Before stool : Irascible irritability.

During stool : Burning, tearing and tenesmus in rectum ;— prolapse of rectum ;—piles ;—rolling in abdomen ;—pallor.

After stool : Pressure in rectum ;—erections ;—lassitude ;— oppression of breath with anxiety; —in epigastrium stitching during pressure.

Calcarea fluorica

Constipation with dizziness and dull headache.

Bleeding piles; tired aching in small of back; itching of anus as from pin worms; crampy, knotting of calves of legs; enlarged veins.

Internal or blind piles frequently, with pain in back, generally far down on the sacrum. Much wind in lower bowels.

Fissure of the anus, and intensely sore crack near the lower end of the bowel.

Calcarea phosphorica

Constipation, with difficult hard stool.

Boils and abscesses about and near the anus, discharging blood and pus.

Sore feeling in anus; worse outside, with a stitching, burning and throbbing. Itching in the anus.

Small furuncle near anus, to the right, with much pain; cannot sit, has to stand, or lie on left side; discharges blood or pus, and remains a painless fistula.

Fistula in ano, alternating with chest symptoms.

Fistula in tubercular subjects.

Fissured anus, with burning stitching pains.

Stitching pain in the anus, with or without haemorrhoids.

Bleeding from the rectum and anus during stool.

Piles : Pain keeps on in bed, is intense on standing, walking and touch, ameliorated heat, general suffering, from every cold change of weather; often itch, burn and discharge of yellow pus.

Protruding piles; stitches in the rectum towards the anus or shooting in the anus; hard stool, with depression of mind, causing headache; with old people.

Calcarea sulphurica.

Inveterate constipation. Difficult stool. Inefficient stool. Ineffectual urging to stool. Burning pain during stool. Pain during and after stool. Tenesmus at stool.

The stool is bloody, dry, hard, knotting, large, licentric, soft, white, yellow and purulent.

Painless abscesses of the anus.

Pressing, stitching and soreness in the anus.

Prolapsus of the rectum.

External piles.

Moisture about anus, causing smarting and itching.

Haemorrhage from the rectum and anus.

In the rectum there is formication and intense itching.

Fistula in ano.

Cannabis sativa :

Obstinate constipation ; sometimes causing retention of urine.

Pressure in the rectum and sacral region, as if the intestines were sinking down and would be pressed out, while sitting ; pressure in the rectum towards right side.

Constrictive pains in anus, together with a sensation as if thighs were drawn together.

Sensation, as of a running of cold water from the anus.

Cantharis :

Constipation and hard faeces.

Constipation with retention of urine, or with frequent urination, attended with cutting, burning pains, but little urine passed at a time.

Violent burning in the anus, after the diarrhoea.

Pain in the perineum seemingly arising from the neck of the bladder.

Cutting in the rectum partially relieved by discharge of flatus, entirely relieved by stool.

Passage of pure blood from the anus and urethra.

During stool : Colic, pressing, cutting pains in the anus causing the patient to cry out ;—prolapsus ani.

After stool : Cutting colic, burning, biting or stinging in anus; chilliness, as if cold water were poured over body.

Capsicum annum :

Stool mucous, frequent, mucous mingled with blood, causing tenesmus after drinking. After every stool thirst and after every drink shivering.

Haemorrhoids : Burning, swollen, itching, throbbings; cutting and smarting during defecation, even when the stool is liquid with sore feeling in anus ; bleeding or blind ; with mucous discharge ; profuse flow of blood.

Tenesmus ani, only relieved by squatting down on his heels ; suppressed haemorrhoidal flow, causing me'ancholy ; lack of reactive power, especially in fat, lazy people, easily exhausted and want to lie down constantly.

Varices bleed a long time; the flowing of blood causes a burning pain in the anus; the stool is mixed with bloody mucous; there are drawing pains in the back and cutting pains in the belly.

Before stool : Flatulent colic.

During stool : Burning or biting, stinging in anus—straining; twisting, cutting pain about the navel.

After stool : Straining; thirst.

Carbo animalis :

Stool hard, lumpy, scanty.

Unsuccessful desire for stool; passes only offensive flatus ; pain in the back, and feeling across abdomen, as if there was no expulsive power.

Stool scanty, delayed. Soft stool. Passage of blood during stool.

Oozing of a thin, inodorous fluid from the rectum (also from perinaeum), weak digestion, especially in nursing women, coldness about stomach, by pressing firmly with the hand or by friction.

Burning and soreness in rectum and anus, in the evening.

Piles burning in rectum, in evening; on walking; much swollen.

Fissura-ani, with severe burning.

Discharges are ichorous; but the discharge from piles in incdorous.

Many symptoms occur during menses; headache; itching burning soreness and smarting at vulva and anus ; haemorrhoids.

Before stool : Rigours about the head ;—colicky pains ;—bearing down toward the os pubis; drawing from anus through vulva.

During stool : Stitches in and about the groins ;—cutting pain in haemorrhoids ;—leaving in abdomen proceeding upwards from the vulva ;—backache ;—bloatedness.

After stool : Scratching in rectum ;—weakness and twisting feeling in the bowels ;—rigours ;—desire to urinate, with exhaustion sleepiness without sleep ;—ringing in the ears, and shaking chills.

Carboneum sulphuratum :

Constipation with much belching; difficult stool; ineffectual urging; insufficient stool.

Pain in the rectum after stool ; during stool.

Burning during stool; after stool.

Itching at anus in the morning.

Eruptions about the anus.

Excoriations at anus and between the nates.

Formication in the anus.

Moisture at the anus, itching and burning.

Stitching pain in anus ; evening ; during stool ; cramping stitching in anus and neck of bladder to urethra during urination.

Tenesmus during stool.

Constant prolapsus of rectum.

Haemorrhage of bright red blood.

Haemorrhoids ; bluish ; chronic ; external ; large ; during menses ; very sore ; inactivity of the rectum.

Cutting and pressing outward.

Fistula in ano.

Carbo vegetabilis :

Ineffectual urging to stool. Stool solid and enveloped in mucous.

Before stool much pressure with, at same time, pressure on the bladder and in the back (frequent in women) ; at last with pains like labour-pains, and great straining ; a soft stool.

Itching and burning, stiches and cutting at stool.

In the rectum and anus, burning, both independently of and during the evacuation of flatus and stool.

Discharge of an acrid, corrossive, viscid humour from the anus causing much itching and some smarting, oozing of moisture upon the perinaeum, with soreness and much itching pains in the small of back, burning and tearing in the limbs ; constipation, with burning stools and discharge of blood ; frequent tendency of the blood to the head, flatulence, slow action of the bowels ; epistaxis ; dysuria ; for debauchees ; used-up people, profound adynamia.

Haemorrhoids ; protrude ; blue ; suppurating and emitting a terrible smell ; burning in the rectum ; oozing of humour from the rectum ; flatulence.

(A carbon ointment, made by carbonising a wine cork by plunging it into a clear fire and then, in its still glowing state, into vaseline and mixing thoroughly is regarded as a sovereign remedy in anal irritation and haemorrhoidal troubles).

Many symptoms occur during menses ; headache ; itching, burning soreness and smarting at vulva and anus ; haemorrhoids.

Before stool : Cutting and drawing in abdomen.

During stool : Burning and cutting in anus ; stitches in rectum epistaxis.

After stool : Burning in anus ; straining in the back, rectum and bladder, feeling of emptiness; jamming or pinching stitches in abdomen, bloatedness ; trembling weakness, anxiety with trembling feeling and involuntary motion.

Cardus marianus.

Inveterate constipation.

Stool : black ; hard and knotty, clay like, bileless.

Burning pain in rectum and anus which interferes with sitting.

Haemorrhoids with acidity of stomach and distension of bowels.

Piles : itching ; bleeding.

Carlsbad.

Faeces held back. Stool slow, and only passed by much abdominal pressure.

Burning in rectum with constant pressure ; the rectum is often pressed out.

Shooting pain in rectum and anus frequently extending to penis.

Discharge of bloody mucus with itching and burning in anus extending up towards rectum.

Discharge of blood in drops or in a stream even without stool when walking.

Lumps as larger as hazel nuts at anus, with burning after stool and impeded walking.

Bleeding piles.

Cascarilla :

Profuse bright blood with or without stool, in large quantities, causing weakness ; diarrhoea alternating with hard lumpy stool ; constant slight urging, often with pain high up in rectum.

Causticum :

Stool : soft and small, size of goose-quill. Hard, tough, covered with mucus ; shines like greese ; small-shaped ; expelled with much straining, or only on standing up. Partial paralysis of rectum.

Frequent loud emission of offensive flatus. Pressure in the rectum. Itching in the anus and genitals. Pain in the perinaeum with pulsation.

After evacuation, anguish, with palpitation of the heart and burning in the anus.

Haemorrhoids impending the stool, swollen, itching, stitching, stinging, burning like fire, painful when touched ; pain increased when walking, standing, when thinking of them, accompanied with obstinate constipation, with ineffectual urging.

Frequent, sudden pressive, penetrating pain in rectum.

Useful for clergymen (and public speakers) who have an attack of piles after every effort to preach or straining the voice.

Excoriates between nates from walking or sitting.

The haemorrhoids become infiltrated and hardened.

Fissures which tend to dry up and have dark brown or purple edge ; walking causes pain in and bleeding from anus.

Large painful pustule near the anus, discharging pus, blood and serum.

Pressure in the haemorrhoidal tumours of the rectum, so as to cause them to protrude.

Before stool : Anxiety ;—twisting abdominal pains.

During stool : Discharge of mucous.

After stool : Biting and burning in anus ; pinching in the hypochondria ; anxiety with heat of the face, nausea ; running of water from the mouth.

Chamomilla :

Bleeding piles with colic, with compressive pain in the abdomen, frequent urging to stool, occasional burning and corrosive diarrhoeic stools ; tearing pain in the small of the back, worse at night.

Ulcerating fissures at the anus; great restlessness, crying, screaming, tossing ; sweating ; angry, peevish and ill-humoured.

Chelidonium majus :

Constipation, stool hard, in hard lumps.

Periodic straining and pressing on rectum, as if before a stool without result.

Burning ; cutting ; drawing ; crawling and itching ; sticking and itching in rectum and anus (Haemorrhoids).

Some blood with stool.

Chimaphila umbellata :

Inclination to stool, either ineffectual or attended with great pain.

Obstinate constipation, with haemorrhoids.

China officinalis :

Constipation ; large accumulation ; stool difficult, even if soft ; after long purging.

Pressure and shootings in the rectum and the anus.

In the rectum stitches, also during stool. Tingling in the anus.

Mucous discharge from the rectum.

Bleeding piles ; burning and burning-itching ; tingling in the anus with creeping (crawling, as of worms) and itching, extending into urethra, attended with burning in the glans.

Before stool : Colic.

During stool : Stitches and acrid feeling in anus ;—thirst.

After stool: Renewed desire ;—creeping in rectum as if caused by worms ;—headache ;—stiffness in the nape of neck ;—backache ;—exhaustion.

Chinninum arsenicosum :

Constipation, with hard, knotty stools.

Involuntary stool and urine.

Pain in the anus during stool.

Burning in the anus during diarrhoea, during stool. Pressing pain. Stitching. Itching.

Paralytic weakness of the rectum. Ineffectual urging to stool.

Moisture about the anus.

Bleeding from anus ; haemorrhoids.

Chininum sulphuricum :

At the anus, sensation of the heat extending to the other intestines.

Prolapse of rectum, especially in children.

Increases of haemorrhoidal phenomena, itching at the rectum and tenesmus.

Flowing of arterial blood from the anus ; bloodly flux from the rectum.

Chromicum acidum :

Blind piles, with costiveness.

External piles disappeared, became internal and bleeding,

Copious discharge of haemorrhoidal blood ; with weakness in back.

Cimex :

Stools hard, in small balls.

After the discharge of a small piece of white stool the rectum closes firmly.

Stools with haemorrhoidal sufferings ; pain during stool.

Cinnabaris :

Obstinate constipation, stools hard and too large.

Protrusion of anus during stool.

Sensation of formication in the anus, as if from a large worm.

Little pimples around the anus, with burning and itching ; thin stools and tenesmus.

Bleeding piles.

Clematis erecta :

Hard stool, difficult to discharge (in the evening).

Haemorrhoids, itching, dicharging some mucus.

Before stool : Colic.

During stool : Burning in rectum ; swelling of piles ; heat.

After stool : Alleviation of bloatedness and headache ; itching anus ; burning in anus.

Cocculus indicus :

Evacuation hard and difficult.

Ineffectual desire for stool, with constipation ; tenesmus.

Contractive pain in the rectum, preventing sitting (in the afternoon).

Many symptoms are worse at menstrual period ; piles during menses.

Before stool : Colic.

After stool : Straining in rectum ; faintness.

(The weaker and the more nervous the woman the more liable to be COCCULUS. Nausea and distressing vertigo acpcomany nearly all diseases needing COCCULUS).

Colchicum autumnale :

During stool sensation as if the sphincter ani were torn to pieces. Cramps in the sphincter ani.

Tingling itching, burning, and tearing in the anus.

Protrusion of rectum.

Before stool : Feeling like diarrhoea in anus ;—flatulence ; pinching in the abdomen.

During stool : Stinking flatus ;—rending pain in anus ;—backache ;—vomiting, vertigo, faintness, cardial stitches.

After stool : Remission of intestinal pains and of sensorial complaints ;—increase of pelvic pains ;—stinking flatus, feeling of diarrhoea in rectum, and sore biting in anus ;—renewed desire to go to stool.

Collinsonia canadensis :

Constipation, stools light coloured and lumpy, with hard straining, followed by dull pains in the anus and hypogastrium ; stool in form of balls. (COLLINSONIA inclines more toward constipation, ALOES to diarrhoea.)

Tendency to flatulent colic ; alternation of haemorrhoidal suffering (with suppressed haemorrhoidal bleeding) with cerebral and cardiac troubles (dilated right heart) ; haemorrhoids during or as a sequela of pregnancy and parturition, with constipation and malposition or prolapsus uteri. It has cured inveterate cases of dyspepsia with weight in epigastrium and piles.

Piles during catamenia. Prolapse of the rectum with piles.

Chronic, painful, bleeding piles, though not profusely or protruding piles with bleeding ; sensation of the rectum as if sticks, Sand or gravel had lodged there; grow worse as evening approaches till late at night, better in the morning, constipation of the bowels and pain in the epigastrium, with loss of appetite ; or diarrhoea.

Most of the symptoms of COLLINSONIA are due to protal congestion and hence it is such an important haemorrhoidal remedy—in fact no remedy can equal COLLINSONIA in obstinate cases of haemorrhoids which bleed almost incessantly. We think of this remedy, especially in the chronic variety of piles with heavy ache in the pelvis and a great itching and burning in the anus with a certain amount of prolapsus.

The patient complains of great uneasiness, weight, pressure and pain in the rectum. The patient is prostrated due to great and continuous loss of blood. *Dull pain in the head with constipation*, and the association of *headache with haemorrhoidal conditions* are two very characteristic features of COLLINSONIA to be always borne in mind. Passed blood in the stools; the heart symptoms coming on when the bleeding ceased and disappeared when it was re-established.

Colocynthis :

Constipation, and evacuations retarded (during pregnancy). During the evacuation, contraction in the rectum.

Painful swelling of the haemorrhoidal tumours of the anus, and of the rectum.

Terrible colic, causing cramping up double and great restlessness from on account of haemorrhoids.

Pricking at anus with constant discharge of mucus. Burning and darting pains at anus.

Blood flows continuously and for a long time from piles with violent sticking, stitching, and burning pains in small of back and anus.

Paralysis of the sphincter ani.

During stool : Flatus, colic, nausea, feeling of coldness.

After stool : Remission of colic ;—distension ;—lassitude.

Conium maculatum :

Frequent ineffectual urging to stool; or small quantity passed each time.

After the evacuations, weakness, palpitation of the heart, frequent expulsion of flatulence, and trembling.

Often more than diarrhoea is constipation with the ineffectual urging, hard stool, paralysis of the rectum.

Inability to strain at stool, inability to expel contents because of the paralytic weakness of all the muscles that take part in expulsion.

Constipation with tenesmus. Hard evacuations, only every second day.

Heat and burning sensation in the rectum, while evacuating and at other times ; frequent stitching in the anus.

Emission of foetid or cold flatulence ; (stool feels cold).

Faeces, with streaks of blood.

Copaiva officianalis :

Insufficient stools ; stools like sheep's dung.

Stools with tenesmus ; bloody stools.

Stitching spasms in rectum ; intolerable burning and itching at anus.

Fluent piles.

Crocus sativa :

Creeping in the anus, as from ascarides.

Obtuse shooting in the side, and above the anus.

Stitches, tingling and itching at the anus. (stitch extending from the anus through the small of the back into the left groin, increasing during an inspiration.)

Sensitive, dull long stitch near left side of anus, from time to time.

Intolerable writhing in the anus.

Stool contain dark, stringy blood.

Crotalus horridus :

Constipation with congestion to head and headache.

White stools.

Vomiting, purging and micturition simultaneously caused by spasmodic contractions with tenesmus and strangury.

Haemorrhoids, great tendency to bleed, on straining a little at stool, or on standing ; in pregnant women ; with menstrual irregularities ; with heart or liver diseases, in inebriats.

Haemorrhage, dark, fluid, uncoagulable.

Cyclamen europeum :

Urging to stool ; tenesmus.

Drawing, pressive pain in and about the anus and peri-naeum, as if a spot was suppurating, when walking or sitting.

Pressure in rectum or anus.

Heat in rectum, with swelling of the haemorrhoidal veins.

Haemorrhoidal flow.

Before stool : Nausea ; rumbling and pinching in abdomen.

During stool : Straining and burning in anus ;—colic ; palpitation.

After stool : Ineffectual straining at stool ; pinching in abdomen, dullness and forgetfulness.

Derris pinnata :

Sensation of foreign body in anus.

Burning or sharp pains with bloody stool.

Dioscorea villosa :

Black, hard, dry, lumpy stool, last part of it soft, white and mushy, followed by prolapsus.

Itching in the rectum.

Piles like grapes or red cherries, around the anus, not bleeding.

Darting pain, from old haemorrhoidal tumour, to the liver.

Haemorrhoidal tumours of livid colour prolapsed, with great pain and distress in them.

Elaps corallinus :

Crawling at anus as if from worms.

Discharge of black, liquid blood from the bowels and at stool with colic and sensation as if the bowels were twisted.

Constriction of the sphincter ani, after bloody stool.

Prolapsus ani.

Electricitas :

Violent pressure in the rectum (during the stool).

Burning in anus.

Haemorrhoidal flux.

Erigeron canadense :

Stools : Small streaked with blood ; tormina ; burning in the bowels and rectum ; hard lumps of faeces mixed with the discharges.

Haemorrhoids bleeding ; with hard lumpy stools ; burning in the margin of the anus, it feels as if torn.

Haemorrhage from the bowels ; anus-bright redness of the discharge.

Eryngium aquaticum :

Constipation : Stools dark leaden colour, dry and very hard ; tenesmus at stool with a sensation of cutting as they pass through anus.

Haemorrhoids and prolapsus ani.

Euphrasia officinalis :

Old flat condylomata at the anus, with severe burning ; worse at night.

Pressure in the anus while sitting ; even in piles.

Cough after the disappearance of haemorrhoids.

Before stool : Flatus.

After stool : Burning in anus ;—feeling of warmth.

Ferrum metallicum :

Costive ; stools hard and difficult, followed by backache or cramping pain in rectum ; ineffectual urging ; itching of anus as from ascarides, especially in young children.

Protrusion of large piles, worse at rest.

Blind and fluent haemorrhoids, copious bleeding or ichorous oozing ; tearing pains with itching and gnawing.

Prolapsus recti ; with children.

Before stool : Flatulency :—paleness of the face.

During stool : Cramp-like pain in abdomen, back, and anus ; pains in the stomach.

After stool : Lassitude.

Ferrum muriaticum :

Obstinate constipation.

Dry cough, ending in retching ; itching of nose and anus, enuresis, headache, neuralgia, nervousness.

Ascarides coincident with bleeding piles.

Ferrum phosphoricum :

Constipation, with heat in the lower bowel, associated with prolapse and haemorrhoids and aversion to meat diet, difficult stool ; constriction of anus.

Involuntary stools. Catarrh of stomach and bowels.

Pain in rectum ; during stool ; with dysentery, and fever ; from inflammation, constant aggravation by pressure of stomach.

Disposition to prolapsus recti. Prolapsus of anus, during stool.

Haemorrhoids, inflamed or bleeding ; bright-red blood with a tendency to coagulate, before any induration occurs ; external piles.

Fluoricum acidum :

Soft small stools in the morning after drinking coffee, and again in the evening, with protrusion of haemorrhoids.

Protrusion of the anus during an evacuation.

The itching of the anus is sometime intense; profuse haemorrhage after stool; itching around and in anus, in perinaeum.

Constipation with piles.

Before stool : Stinking flatus;—abdominal pain.

During stool : Burning and protrusion of anus or piles ;— pinching abdominal pain.

After stool : Tenesmus; abdominal pain.

Gambogia :

Hard, insufficient stool, with violent urging and pressing succeeded by burning at the anus.

Diarrhoea, with burning pain and tenesmus of the rectum, prolapsus ani, and constant pinching around the umblicus, sometimes atteneded with discharge of mucus.

Gastein :

Constipation and moving of flatulence in abdomen, with ineffectual desire in rectum; very hard stool.

Feeling of contraction in rectum.

Bleeding haemorrhoids.

Graphites :

Constipation; large knotty faeces; chronic, with hardness in region of liver. After stool, there is some mucus remaining about the anus.

Protrusion of rectum, without urging to stool, as if the anus were lame. The rectum seems to have lost its contractile power, and the varices protrude.

Large haemorrhoidal tumours, varices of the rectum and burning rhagades between them.

Haemorrhoids, with pain on sitting down, or on taking a wide step, as if split with a knife, also violent itching, and very sore to touch.

Fissures of recent origin, especially in children; fissura ani; severe, sharp, cutting pain during stool, followed by constriction and aching for several hours, worse at night.

"From the anus there is copious discharge of very offensive flatus day and night. While diarrhoea is not so common as constipation yet it is a marked condition in some patients. With the loose stools, and with the constipated stools copious white jelly-like mucus is often found. Discharge of mucus from anus and a constant moisture about the outside parts. Long narrow stools. It has cured many cases of bleeding piles of long standing where there was extreme soreness and fissures and great burning. No desire to go to stools for many days. Eczema and herpes near the anus or involving anus. Now if all this should occur in subjects of this tendency to sticky eruptions, we should not hesitate to give GRAPHITES with expectations of success."

"In eczematous subjects where the anus is extremely sore and the stools are covered with mucus, with no tenesmus or constriction. Chronic constipation, with hardness in hepatic region; moist humid eruption on scalp and behind ears; watery leucorrhoea at the time of menstruation; scanty and delayed menses; piles accompanied by dizziness."

Before stool : Loathing and pains in abdomen.

During stool : Straining and burning in anus.

After stool : Distension, uneasiness, and pinching in abdomen.

Gratiola officianalis :

Constipation with gouty acidity.

Stools with burning and protrusion of large stinging and a burning tumours. Passage of faeces without being conscious of it.

Pain, as from excoriation in the rectum. Burning pain in rectum, during and after the evacuation. Shootings, itching, smarting, and throbbing in the anus. Rectum constricted.

Blind haemorrhoids, haemorrhoids with hypochordriasis.

"Constipation, difficult stools. External piles from any exertion and after stool. Biting, stinging tension in tumours. During stool, a sensation as if the rectal membrane was torn. After stool, all the nerves of the pelvis seem in a high state of tension, the flesh on the perinaeum feels as if torn from the bone. Sleepless before midnight; peevish; melancholy."

Hamamelis virginica :

Stools : Costive; hard, coated with mucus. Large quantities of a tar-like blood.

Varices protrude through   the anus and the haemorrhoidal. Veins, look distinctly bluish and distended to fulness, with their contents of venous blood.

Profusely bleeding haemorrhoids, characterised by burning soreness, fulness and weight; at times rawness of the anus; the back feels as if it would break off; pricking pain, worse from pressure, from the wrist to the shoulder along the course of superficial veins; the same pricking pain in the region of the heart; scanty menses.

Haemorrhage from piles, where the loss of a small quantity of blood is followed by prostration out of proportion to the loss of blood.

Venous congestion, haemorrhages, varicose veins, and haemorrhoids with bruised soreness of affected parts, seem to be the special sphere of this remedy. Haemorrhoids, when attended with profuse bleeding at regular intervals and without much expulsive effort,   stand in equal   need of HAMAMELIS. Haematuria and haemorrhoids of the bladder, when characterised by dull pain in the renal and vesical region and associated with constant urging with urination, can be easily checked with HAMAMELIS ; severe frontal headache, restless nights ; pulsation in rectum as if piles would protrude.

Helleborus niger :

Hard, scanty stool, during and immediately after which violent cutting, shooting in rectum, from below up, just as if it contracted tightly, and as if a body with cutting edges struck there.

After an evacuation, burning hot smarting at the anus.

Haemorrhoids.

Before stool : Abdominal pain.

During stool : Cutting stinging in rectum upwards ; nausea and abdominal pain.

After stool : Burning biting anus.

Heloderma :

Stool soft, dark, difficult to expel.

Haemorrhoids swollen, itch and bleed.

Hepar sulphuris calcareum :

Constipation : Stools hard and dry ; especially with eruption in bend of elbows ; or in popliteal space. Faeces not hard, but expelled with difficulty.

Protrusion of haemorrhoids.   Haemorrhage from the rectum, with soft stool.

Haemorrhoids from engorgement of the liver with great abdominal distress, preventing abdominal respiration, abdomen swollen and somewhat tender ; obstinate constipation.

Sensation as if bruised in small of back and thighs ; great want of vital power of expulsion from the congested condition of the veins in rectum.

Inflammation and suppuration of haemorrhoidal tumours. After evacuation, pain, as of excoriation, and sanious discharge from the anus.

Before stool : Pinching in the abdomen.

During stool : Abdominal pain, straining pressing, rumbling and nauseous feeling in abdomen ; heat in hands and cheeks ; inclination to lie down.

After stool : Sore pain in anus and sanious secretion ;— tympanitis ;—obstruction of the nose.

Hydrastis canadensis :

Constipation with a sinking feeling in stomach, and dull headache ; stool lumpy, covered with mucus.

Haemorrhoids, costive ; even a slight haemorrhoidal flow exhausts, contraction and spasm.

Fistula ani.

"Burning and smarting pain in rectum and anus after each stool, lasting for hours, with hot sensation in bowels, colic and faintness ; stools dry, large, lumpy, nodulated; dyspeptic cough with expectoration of ropy mucous. "

Painful piles, severe burning, smarting pains in rectum before and after stool, with paroxysms of headache and constipation ; flatulent colic accompanied by faintness ; catarrh of the bladder, with thick, ropy, mucus sediment in the urine ; faintness, goneness physical prostration ; icterus.

Hyosciamus niger :

Constipation with epilepsy.

Piles bleed profusely; fulness of the veins, full pulse, skin and muscles lax.

During stool : Pain in anus ; flatulency.

After stool : Tiredness.

Hypericum perfoliatum :

Urging, dry, dull, pressing pain.

Haemorrhoids, with pain, bleeding and tenderness.

Piles ; burning, biting, and feeling of dryness in rectum.

Ignatia amara :

Fruitless efforts and urging to stool. Stools large and soft but passed with difficulty. Stitches from the anus up the rectum. Sharp, pressive pain in the rectum.

Prolapsus of the rectum from moderate straining at stool.

Contractive sore pain in the rectum, like from blind haemorrhoids, one or two hours after stool, worse while standing.

Itching and crawling in the rectum, as from thread worms.

Blind haemorrhoids, with pressure and soreness in anus and rectum ; painful sitting and standing less painful when walking though renewed by taking the fresh air.

Bleeding piles ; violent shooting pains high up into the rectum; for quiet people, or such as get easily excited; after confinement.

Spasmodic constriction of anus, strangulating piles; bleeding during and after stool ; haemorrhage and pain worse when stool is loose, pains return at the same hour each day.

Sudden sharp stitches in haemorrhoids, shooting upward into the body with every cough.

Asthmatic symptoms in haemorrhoidal subjects.

Fissura ani ; pruritus ani.

Before stool : Cutting abdominal pains.

During stool : Flatus ; soreness of rectum ard prolapse of the same.

After stool : Contraction of anus; pressing in rectum; painful piles ;—lassitude.

Iodium :

Constipation ; Hard, knotty, dark coloured faeces.

In the evening, sensation of itching and burning in the anus.

Piles protrude and burn ; worse from heat.

Ipecacuanha :

Evacuation of black matter like pitch.

Haemorrhoids bleed profusely.   Itching of anus.

Kali bichromicum :

Constipation ; stool scanty and lump, followed by burning and pressure in the anus.

Burning pain in anus; after stool; in forenoon with pressure.

Sensation of a plug in anus in afternoon when sitting.

Haemorrhoids which protrude after stool which are very painful ; fulness of haemorrhoidal vessels.

Kali bromatum :

Constipation ; stools very dry, hard and infrequent.

During stool : sensation as if bowels were falling out ; dribbling of urine.

Spasmodic stricture of sphincter ani.

Constant diarrhoea and more or less tenesmus, and passage of much blood on making efforts to expel, protrusion of several elongated bodies resembling earthworms ; with this expulsion there was always a yellow, very foetid discharge ; faeces flatened ; flatulent distension of bowels ; patient pale and sickly looking (polypus of rectum).

Blind, intensely painful piles with black stools.

Pain in haemorrhoids, fissure of rectum and painful growths.

Kali carbonicum :

Stool dry, too large in size, rectum inactive feels distressed an hour or two before stool.

In consequence of constipation with too large stools ; the haemorrhoidal tumours swell and become large and very painful ; they bleed.

Sensation as if a red hot poker were being thrust up the rectum, worse by sitting in cold water ; stinging, burning, tearing, itching pain, even after a natural stool, setting patient nearly crazy and depriving him of sleep.

Stool insufficient, soft bloody, like sheep's dung.

Inflammation, soreness, stitches, and tingling as from ascarides, in haemorrhoids. Coughing aggravates pain in haemorrhoids.

Protrusion of haemorrhoids during micturition, emitting first blood, afterwards white mucus.

Haemorrhoids complicating fistula ani, especially in persons suffering from lung troubles.

Sensation as if anus would be fissured, worse by horse back exercise or by any pressure on anus.

"KALI CARB. has a great many complaints of the rectum and anus and of the stool. It has most persistent and enormus haemorrhoidal tumours that burn, that are extremely sensitive to touch, that bleed copiously that are extremely painful, making it impossible for him to sleep. He is compelled to lie upon the back and hold the nates apart, because the pressure is very painful to the external piles. The piles cannot be put back ; there is great distension and swelling in-side. Haemorrhoids that come out after stool and bleed copiously and are very painful ; they must be pushed back and long after going to bed they burn like fire. There is great aggravation from stool, which is hard and knotty and requires great straining to expel. Fistula of the anus. Burning temporarily relieved by sitting in cold water." KENT.

(KALI CARB. cures conditions   due to   psora, or to the suppression of eruptions in childhood, or to the closing up of old ulcers and fistulous openings with a history of troubles ever since. All the wandering pains and chilliness are again relieved by eruptions by the outbreak of discharges, by haemorrhages, by ulcers that eat in deep and flout freely and fistulous openings.)

Kali muriaticum :

Constipation of infants during dentition ; only passing small quantity ; stools knotty, like sheep's dung crumbling at verge of anus.

Painful smarting haemorrhoids.

Haemorrhoids bleeding ; blood dark and thick ; fibrinous, clotted.

Kali phosphoricum :

Constipation with very difficult stool ; hard, large, knotty.

Inactivity of the rectum. Involuntary stool. Pain in rectum during and after stool. Soreness and pressing pain, stitching pains. Tenesmus after stool.

Paralysis of the rectum. Relaxed anus. Ineffectual urging to stool.

The stool is excoriating; bloody mucus or pure blood, brown, clay-coloured, watery stool; putrid flatus followed by tenesmus after breakfast.

Inflamed piles with offensive moisture.

Haemorrhoids protruding, with swelling and burning pains.

Paretic condition of rectum [and colon following removal of haemorrhoids.

Kali sulphuricum :

Constipation that is very obstinate, alternating with diarrhoea.

Stool difficult, soft or hard, insufficient, during menses, from inactivity of the rectum.

Sensation of faintness in stomach and dull feeling in head, fearing to loose her senses.

Involuntary stool, violent itching of the anus.

Pain in the rectum and anus, during stool, after stool; BURNING during diarrhoea, during stool, after stool.

Haemorrhage from the anus.

Haemorrhoids ; external, large and bleeding; with catarrh of stomach and yellow mucus coated tongue.

Lachesis :

Costive, ineffectual urging; anus feels closed. Stools offensive, even if formed.

Tormenting urgency but not to stool. Wants to pass stool, but the pain is so increased thereby he must desist.

Constriction of rectum; anus feels tight as if nothing could go through it.

Burning in anus during and after stools; itching at anus; worse after sleep; beating in the anus as from hammers.

Stool lies close to anus without passing and without urging, spasmodic pain in anus before and after stool; protrusion after stool ; rectum prolapsed and tumefied.

Piles protruding or strangulated, or with stitches upward at each cough or sneeze, worse at climaxis; or with drunkards; with scanty menstrual flow.

Visible spasmodic tenesmus in paroxysms, from two to five minutes, exhorting cries; pass blood and mucus, sometimes with violent colic.

Painful constriction of anus followed by collapse.

Haemorrhoids with colic, or with burning and cutting in rectum, or with congestion of blood in anus and diarrhoea.

Piles irritable, with painful drawing upward like a mouse lugging at one side and drawing it up.

Lactuca virosa

At anus : Drawing; pricking, towards evening (bruised pain); haemorrhoidal tumours round anus, with tenesmus in rectum and a fresh evacuation of a liquid stool after each solid evacuation.

During stool : General lassitude, fatigue so as almost to bring on sleep, yawning, and accumulation of water in mouth.

After stool : (soft), pressure in the anus.

Leptandra virginica :

Constipation and distressing pain beneath the sacrum.

Prolapse of rectum with haemorrhoids.

Frequently bleeding piles.

Lilium tigrinum :

Constipation; hard and dark stools, then heat in rectum and anus and pain in abdomen.

Frequent urging to stool and no stool in the rectum; with a sensation as if a ball were in the rectum.

Haemorrhoids after delivery, sore to touch, itching; bearing down at stool as if all would protrude through vagina.

Most inveterate protruding haemorrhoids with burning.

Lobelia inflata :

Bleeding piles; copious haemorrhage.

Discharge of black blood after stool; debility; sensation of weakness and oppression at the epigastrium, with oppression of chest.

(A few drops of LOB-IN. in boiling water takes away the pain and tension of inflamed piles; the patient sits on a utensil thus filled.)

Lycopodium clavatum :

Constipation; ineffectual urging from the contraction of the sphincter ani.

Discharge of blood, even with soft stool.

Continued burning or stitching pain in the rectum.

Varices protrude painful when sitting.

About the anus, itching and a moist, tender eruption; painful to touch.

Piles which do not mature, but from partial absorption their contents remain as hard, bluish lumps.

Bleeding piles which contain an amount of blood, a far greater quantity of blood than the size of the vein would warrant.

Great tendency to excoriations about anus which bleed easily.

Haemorrhoids swell and protrude and bleed, even when there is no constipation.

Stitching and burning at stool, even when the faeces are not hard.

Aching and pressure in the rectum, especially at night.

Itching and tension at the anus in the evening in bed.

Cutting in the rectum and bladder, long-continued pain after stool.

Distension of the whole abdomen, and rumbling after stool.

"Lycopodium patients are generally costive. They suffer from frequent ineffectual desire for stool. This is not due to irregular peristalisis as in NUX VOM; but to the presence of constriction in rectum. Each evacuation cause terrible amount of pain and urging that leaves the patients in a very prostrated condition. In some bad cases we may notice syncope after the stool. The mucous membrane of the rectum is very much injected, excoriated and is full of numerous haemorrhoidal knobs. The examining finger encounters spasmodic constriction of the sphincter. There is no narrowing of rectum due to the same cause. The most stricking symptom to remember is the persistence of pain after evacuation. It is so severe as to arrest breathing. The pain is cutting, tearing, stitching and cramping in nature".

"It has troublesome haemorrhoids, but they are non-descript. Any kind of haemorrhoids may be cured by LYCOPODIUM, if the flatulence, the stomach symptoms, the mental symptoms, and the general symptoms of LYCOPODIUM are present, because the haemorrhoidal symptoms are numerous."

Lycopus :

Constipation lasting six or seven days, stool dry and clay-like. (Restores haemorrhoidal flow after suppression and relieves other symptoms.)

Magnesia muriatica :

Stools; in large, hard lumps; insufficient; crumbling at verge of anus; abdomen distended; knotty like sheep's dung.

Absence of desire for stool, atony as with the bladder.

Much pressure to stool; violent tenesmus, with scanty evacuation, or only an emission of flatus.

Burning and smarting in anus during and after stool.

Obstruction of bowels from induration of faeces.

Haemorrhoids pain during normal stool.

Mancinella :

Stools; frequent, thin, watery, with vomiting; painful, black, foetid bloody, with tenesmus.

After stool : Pulsation in anus, discharge of foetid blood from piles.

Medorrhinum :

Constriction and inertia of bowels with ball-like stools, round balls, and hard lumpy stool.

Can only pass stool by leaning very far back; very painful, as if there was a lump on posterior surface of sphincter; so painful as to cause tears.

Stool tenacious, clay-like, sluggish, cannot be forced from sensation of prolapsus of rectum.

Profuse bloody discharges from rectum, sometimes in large clotted masses, followed by shivering.

Melilotus alba :

Constipation : No desire for stool till there is a large accumulation, when there is a very difficult, painful stool with constriction in rectum and discharge of stringy glossy, milk-white mucus; each succeeding passage less painful until normal, then constipation sets in again.

Heavy throbbing and fulness in rectum from internal piles.

Severe shooting cutting in rectum while walking better sitting down.

Menyanthes :

Constipation : Hard faeces with pinchings in abdomen. Bleeding, haemorrhoidal tumours.

Mercurius :

Constipation : Stool tenacious or crumbling, discharged only with violent straining; constant, ineffectual urging, worse at night.

Pain in sacrum, as after lying on a hard couch. Great weakness, with ebullition and trembling from the least exertion.

Blood before, during and after, even a hard stool.

Large, bleeding piles during stool, which is watery; haemorrhage from the rectum, during mictruition; falling of the rectum, which is black and bleeding ; inflammation and suppuration of the haemorrhoidal tumours.

Mercurius biniodatus :

Pain in anus as if piles would appear.

Inveterate piles.

Mezereum :

Constipation after confinement. It should be prescribed particularly when the stools are hard as stone and are immense in size. It feels as if they would split the anus open. They are so big that they cannot be expelled wholesale. They keep on coming in sections and exhausts the patient so that she trembles. The stools are preceded by chill and followed by long stitches in the rectum.

During stool prolapsus recti; anus becomes painful and constricted about the fallen rectum. Painful constriction, tearing and drawing at the anus, perineum and through urethra ; fissure of anus.

The rectum and anus are the seat of many characteristic symptoms, stitching, burning, itching. Stitches in rectum upwards (in afternoon). Biting, sore pain in anus on walking and a burning in rectum. Pain in anus and anterior part of penis. Pinching in anus and near anus left side. Crawling in anus; much itching. Tenesmus, 'tearing and drawing in anus and perineum, and through whole urethra. Coldness and shuddering, before and after the evacuation.

Millefolium :

Haemorrhoids, with profuse flow of blood; chronic blemorrhoea from atony of mucus membranes; great pain.

Murex :

Difficult evacuations; constipation, during more than five days.

Pressure in anus, like painful lancinations.

Sensation of heavy weight pressing on rectum; swelling of haemorrhoids.

Muriaticum acidum :

Stool difficult as from inactivity of the bowels. Smarting in rectum and anus with soft stool.

Piles, suddenly in children; protruding, reddish-blue, burning; too sore to bear the least touch.

Haemorrhoids most sensitive to all touch; even sheet of toilet paper is painful.

Haemorrhoides protruding, blue or dark purple, especially in pregnant women or in feeble children who are suffering from gastric atony, muscular debility and threatened marasmus·

Inflammation of the pile tumours, hot and pulsating; must lie with limbs wide apart.

Bleeding piles. Burning and cutting during stool.

Burning after stool, ameliorated by warm applications, aggravated from bathing with cool water.

Rectum prolapses easily, cannot urinate it coming down. Also when wind is passed or bowels move.

Piles like a bunch of grapes which look purple and BURN when touched.

Excoriation of anus. Fissures.

Natrum muriaticum :

Constipation : Obstinate, retention of stool; stools irregular, hard unsatisfactory; during menses; stool in large masses; stool like sheep's dung; from inactivity of rectum; anus contracted or torn, bleeding; smarting, or burning afterwards; stitches in the rectum causing or burning afterwards; stitches in the rectum causing hypochondriasis or ill-humour; great torper without pain; from want of moisture, dryness of mucus linings, with watery secretions in other parts; difficult expulsion fissuring anus with uterine displacements; haemorrhoidal; in Addison's Disease. Stools dry, crumbling.

Tenesmus in the rectum, with discharge of flatus and slime.

The rectum seems constricted, and it is only after great effort that some little hard faeces pass which tear the anus so that it bleeds and smarts; and then comes some dirty water.

Varices, painful, stinging and humid; protrusion of the rectum; smarting and beating in the rectum: burning at the anus; herpes on the boundaries of the hair in the nape of the neck; cutting pain in the urethra after micturition.

Piles sting, ooze glutinous fluid; herpetic eruption about the anus.

Constipation is marked by a decided aggravation of all the usual ill-hour.

Natrum sulphuricum :

Hard, knotty stools, streaked with blood accompanied and preceded by smarting in the anus; often with scanty menses.

Difficult expulsion of soft stool.

Emission of foetid flatus in large quantities.

Constant uneasiness in bowels and urging to stool.

Knotty wart-like eruption on the anus and between the thighs.

Itching and crawling in the anus.

Ulceration of rectum with copious bleeding.

Bleeding piles.

Nitricum acidum :

Bowels constipated. Inactivity and inability to evacuate faeces. Pain as if rectum would be torn as under during stool.

No remedy has more decided action upon the anus, and one very characteristic symptom is, "great pain after passage of stool, even soft stool." He walks the floor in agony of pain for an hour or two after a stool. Another very characteristic of this remedy in all these affection is 'pricking pain as of a splinter in the part.

Great straining, but little passes. Rectum feels torn.

Haemorrhages from bowels. Profuse, bright.

Haemorrhoids; protruding, swollen; bleeding; painless or burn ing.

Itching in the anus and rectum.

Moisture and soreness about the anus.

Piles.   Old, pendulous, ceased bleeding, but pain touched, worse in warm weather.

Fissure in rectum; tearing, spasmodic symptoms during stool.

(Selects for its special seat of action the outlets of the body where the mucous membrane and skin meet.)

"Anus excoriated, burning, fissured, covered with warts. Membrane comes with the stool. Much pure blood with the stool not even clotted, very offensive. Ineffectual urging to stool. Sensation as if rectum were filled and he cannot expel it, constipation, painful, hard, difficult stool. Drawing, cutting and pressing before stool ; constant fruitless urging. During stool there is colic, tenesmus, spasmodic constriction of anus, unsatisfactory straining. Splinters in rectum. After stool there is still urging, exhaustion; soreness of anus ; cutting pain ; burning and shooting in rectum ; constriction of anus ; great nervous excitement ; palpitation. The pain keeps her in bed for hours after every stool. Itching and burning in anus. Constant acrid moisture about the anus. Periodical bleeding of rectum and pain in sacrum. Fissures of anus. Painful prolapsus of rectum. This has been most useful remedy in fistula, fissures, condylomata, polypi, carbuncles, cancer of the rectum and haemorrhoids—when the symptoms agree. It has cured carbuncles so sensitive that the patient would cry out when they are touched. Haemorrhoids that are exquisitively painful to touch and at stool; that bleed, external or internal, with burning and sticking during stool. Piles that ulcerate and discharge copiously of blood and pus.

When piles are so painful that she breaks out in sweat, becomes anxious, and pulsated all over, on the slightest touch or at stool, this remedy has been useful. Another important point is the discharge of a foetid watery substance from the anus that keeps it constantly moist."

Nux moschata :

Faintness during or after stool is a great indication.

It is also a haemorrhoidal and haemorrhagic remedy. Protruding piles.

Nux vomica :

Constipation : With rush of blood to the head; with ineffectual urging; obstructed portal circulation: feeling as if part remained unexpelled; stool may be in hard masses; irregular peristalic action, hence frequent ineffecual desire or passing but small quantities at each attempt.

Absence of all desires for defecation is a contra-indication.

Alternate constipation and diarrhoea—after abuse of purgatives.

Haemorrhoids blind or flowing irregular piles; frequent tendency of the blood to the head or abdomen, with distension of the epigastrium and hypochondria; worse from high living or sedantary habits; with burning and sticking in rectum; anus burning; smarting as if cut, some hours after stool. Tearing in anus; constriction after mental exertion, after eating.

Itching blind haemorrhoids, with ineffectual urging to stool ; very painful, after drastic drugs.

Itching in anus with sore pain, as from haemorrhoids.

Discharge of bright red blood with faeces, with sensation of constriction and contraction of rectum. Jerking in anus when not at stool.

If the haemorrhoids be large and blind, with a burning, stinging and constricted feeling in the rectum and a bruised pain in the small of the back, and especially if excited by purgative medicines and external and internal allopathic treatment in persons of sedentary habits or addicted to the use of coffee, wine, liquors, spices etc. NUX VOM. may be prescribed with confidence. Itching haemorrhoids keeping the sufferer awake at night; relieved by cold water or bleeding piles with constant urging to stool, and a feeling as if the bowel would empty itself are further indications.

Haematuria from a suppressed haemorrhoidal flow or menses; ischuria, suppression of urine; backache, must sit up to turn in bed; strangulated piles. Bloodless piles in hysteric women.

"As a general rule, NUX VOMICA is better adapted to the inhabitants of elevated, dry and warm regions, than to the inhabitants of valleys, or of cold and damp countries; all this is the opposite of ARSENIOUS ACID". TESTE.

Paeonia :

Burning in anus after stool; then internal chilliness.

Piles; anus fissured, pain intolerable during and after stool; surrounding purple and covered with thick crusts; ulclers, cracks and rhagades. Ulcers, painful, round sharp-cut edges, exude much moisture.

Fissures, much oozing, atrocious pains during and after stool, prevents sleep, must walk the floor all night.

Biting, itching in anus; orifice swollen.

Fistula ani, diarrhoea with anal burning and internal chilliness.

Burning and biting lasting several hours after stool.

The anus is offensively moisture and sore, smarts all the time.

"On the verge and entrance of the rectum, there were several fissured ulcers with elevated and indurated edges."

PAEONIA is mostly useful in anal abscesses, fissures, fistula and boils.

Petroleum :

Piles and fissures of the anus; great itching; scurf on borders of anus. Excrescences on and in the anus, moist, irregular.

Burning and itching in the anus; tiltilating and smarting; itching herpes on the perineum.

Fissures with diarrhoea; herpes and small boils around and at the verge of the anus.

Piles with great itching, worse at night from heat of bed; from rubbing or scratching.

Phosphoricum acidum :

Protrusion of haemorrhoidal tumours from rectum during stool.

After stool tenesmus; sickening pain about navel.

Tearing, smarting, and itching in anus and rectum.

Itching prick on outer circumference of anus.

Bleeding piles, with intolerable pains while sitting with cramps of upper arm, forearm and wrist.

Phosphorous :

Constipation : Stool long, narrow, like a dog's, tough and hard voided with difficulty; white hard stools.

Paralysis of lower bowels and sphincter ani. Anus feels as if wide open.

Needle-like stitches in rectum when not at stool; burning in rectum and anus with great exhaustion; tearing in rectum; and genitals, even to sinking down.

Darting and shakings in rectum and anus (this may occur in children, causing them to cry out, is usually worse in evening or night; they appear to have worms; they will put their hands to the seat, and show by various signs where and what the matter is).

Discharge of mucus out of the gaping anus; stinging or itching at anus; worse evening and night, when lying on back or left side; better when lying right side, from rubbing or after sleeping.

Bleeding piles, with severe lancinating pains; blood flows with each stool in small stream; ulceration of the rectum, with discharge of blood and pus; discharge of dark coagulated blood; verigo, especially on looking up or down.

It has many times cured bleeding, protruding haemorrhoids, haemorrhoids that burn; polypi of the rectum; inflammation of the rectum.

Pain in anus so violant it seemed as though the body would be torn asunder. With cutting and movements in whole abdomen, constant ineffectual desire for stool, heat in hands and anxiety; better only by application of warm clothes.

Fissure of anus.

Physostigma :

Constipation; from atony.

Tenesmus and burning, with diarrhoea; also tenesmus of bladder.

Stool irregular and loose, anus sore and inclined to protrude; piles (absent for three years) return.

Sphincter ani, swollen and rigid, evacuation painful: rectum protruding, swollen and very sensitive.

Severe piles following childbirth.

Phytolacca decandra :

Constipation: Habitual; of the aged, or of those with weak heart; the patient says the bowels will not move without the aid of purgatives; feeling of fulness, in abdomen before stool, which remains after stool, as if all had not passed; from torpor of the rectum; hard stools.

Neuralgic pains in anus and lower part of rectum, shooting along perineum to middle of penis; in the middle of night (with constipation).

Heat in rectum with burning in stomach.

Bleeding piles; bloody discharge with heat in rectum.

Haemorrhoids, permanent and obstinate; bleeding and mucus.

Ulceration; fissure.

Pinus sylvestris :

Constipation; stool, thin, pasty, with colic and great excitement; bilious.

Discharge of round worms ; itching and burning on anus; bloody, slimy, haemorrhoidal discharge for several days.

Platinum metallicum :

Constipation. After lead poisoning or while travelling; sometimes very obstinate; the stool is discharged with difficulty, seeming to stick to anus and rectum like putty.

Frequent itching, tingling, and tenesmus in anus especially in the evening (before sleep). Violent and dull lancinations in rectum.

Hysterical and haemorrhoidal subjects.

Plumbum metallicum :

Painful retraction and constriction of anus. Intolerable pain from spasms of rectum with every evacuation lasting an hour or two, horrible constriction, much worse if stool solid.

Prolapsus ani, with paralysis.

Fissures of anus.

Podophyllum :

Constipation ; clay-coloured, hard dry, difficult ; with flatulence and headache.

Piles with prolapsus ani and long-standing diarrhoea, worse morning.

Prolapsus ani, with stool, even with least exertion, following stool, or thick, transparent mucus, or mixed with blood.

With the stool there is very commonly a prolapse of the rectum; a gush of watery stool and a prolapse of the rectum; a soft stool with great straining and a prolapse of the rectum.

Protrusion of rectum after stool or any sudden motion such as sneezing and mental excitement, sometimes prolapsed for days owing to swelling and congestion.

Faintness, with sensation of emptiness in abdomen, after stool.

"Stools yellow, green or brownish and watery; mucus streaked with blood ; and these attended with heat in the rectum, by flashes of heat running up the back, by painful tenesmus, and by a descent of the rectum. Hence a valuable remedy in dysentery, especially when the patient complaints of a sensation of weakness in the rectum. This prolapsus is to be distinguished from that of IGN., CARB-VEG. and HAM., in that it occurs before the evacuation of faeces and not after it. The anus is extremely sore. From these symptoms we might gather that PODOPHYLLUM would be a valuable remedy in prolapsus ani following dysentery in haemorrhoids."

Psorinum :

Hard, difficult stool, with blood from rectum and burning piles; soreness in rectum and anus when riding; itching in anus.

Burning haemorrhoidal tumours; large quantities of blood from rectum; pain in small of back.

Pulsatilla :

Obstinate constipation, nauseous, bad taste in morning, must wash out her mouth; costive stools hard and large, after suppressed intermittent fever by quinine. Desire for stool, insufficient or no evacuation of faeces, but instead yellowish, sometimes blood mixed with mucus.

Blind haemorrhoids, with itching and sticking pains; painful protruding, blind piles, with stitches, smarting, and soreness. Pressure in rectum after stool.

Blind and flowing haemorrhoids; discharge of blood and slime with the stool; colicky pain; painful pressure upon the haemorrhoidal tumours; backache, fainting spells, mild, gentle and tearful disposition, dryness and bad taste in the mouth every morning ; no thirst.

Violent pains in the haemorrhoids, worse lying down, ameliorated by gentle motion, worse from the warmth of bed, better moving about in the open air. She becomes so nervous in a room while at rest that the pains seem intensified and she must move about.

> "PULSATILLA is one of the best remedies in haemorrhoids after AESCULUS. Passive congestion and dyspeptic troubles are the key-notes. It acts best in the higher potencies."

Piles (blind) with menses; though generally with this remedy, they bleed.

Ranunculus scelleratus :

Itching, tickling, burning of anus; moisture in anus; fine stitches into rectum.

Great urging after a meal; only flatus passes.

Itching and pressing out sensation at anus, as if premonitory of haemorrhoids, worse walking.

Ratania :

RATANIA is said to meet more rectal cases than any other remedy.

Protrusion of the varices after hard stool, with straining and violent pressing in the rectum; burning at the anus before and during a diarrhoeic stool.

Burning in anus like fire, preceding and accompanying defecaction and lasting a long time after, accompanied by protrusion of varices; dry heat in anus, with sudden stitches like stabs with a penknife ; sensation as if the rectum protruded and went back with a jerk, with most horrible pains ; frequent and ineffectual desire to urinate ; burning in urethra while urinating.

> "The sphere in which its efficacy has been mostly demonstrated is the fissure of the anus. The patient suffers the agonies of death. The anus burns like fire, not only during defecation but also before and after. After each stool he feels as if splinters of glass were sticking in every direction in anus and rectum. Sometimes the straining for stool is so very great that defecation is accompanied by protrusion of haemorrhoids. This burning for hours after each stool is a characteristic symptom, and is only relieved by the application of hot water. There is a quite bit of constricting sensation in the rectum. The stools are forced with great effort and the anus aches and burns for hours after the stool."

Fissures : Of anus ard nipples ; of anus, great constriction, terrible pain after stool, especially burning like fire.

> "The burning persisting for a long time after the stool is a very characteristic of RATANIA."

Bursting headache accompanies and follows a straining at stool.

Rhus toxicodendron :

Before stool a burning in the rectum. After stool all pains are relieved. Itching and burning in rectum, with smarting, blind haemorrhoids.

Labour-like drawing towards the uterus, when standing; pain in the small of the back, as if bruised, when lying or sitting still, going off when moving about.

Sense of constriction in rectum, as though one side had grown up.

Sore, blind haemorrhoids, protruding after stool, with pressing in the rectum, as if everything would come out, at night, from cold, pressure, rest.

Haemorrhage of black blood from the bowels.

Fissures of the anus, with periodical profuse bleeding from the anus; sore piles protruding after stool, drawing in the back, from above downward, pain in the small of the back as if bruised, when keeping quiet; frequent urging to urinate, day and night, with increased secretion.

Rumex crispus :

Constipation for several days, followed by a dry, hard stool.

Itching at anus with discharge of offensive flatus.

Sensation as from pressure of a rough stick forced up rectum, painful on walking.

Haemorrhoids protrude; much heat and itching at anus, and sensation as if a foreign body there.

Ruta graveolens :

Stool : Soft discharge with difficulty, from inactivity of the rectum; rectum protrudes immediately on attempting a passage; lumpy slimy; or bloody with much flatus; seemingly only flatus; empty eructations, distended abdomen; faeces often escape when bending over.

Frequent unsuccessful urging, with prolapsus ani.

Constipation, alternating with mucus frothy stools.

Prolapsus of the rectum immediately on attempting a passage. It comes out on the least straining and even from the slightest stooping.

Pain in the rectum when sitting. Nausea felt in rectum.

Great soreness in rectum as from ulceration; dischaige of blood with stool; pruritus ani with smooth appearance of skin round anus.

"RUTA is a good remedy for prolapsus after confinement."

"A useful remedy in piles and stricture of the rectum."

Sabina :

Sense of fulness.   Constipation.

Discharge of sanguineous mucus from anus; blood after a hard evacuation.

Haemorrhoids, with discharge of bright red blood or blood and mucus, causing pain in back, from sacrum to pubis, followed by great lassitude and heaviness.

Painful haemorrhoidal pimples in anus, tingling in anus.

Sangunaria :

Constipation; stools in hard lumps; ineffectual desire with sensation of thick mass in lower part of rectum, repeated several times in the day without stool, and discharge of offensive flatus only.

Haemorrhoids, distressing, cutting, spasmodic, sensation in evening ; recurred several days.

Sepia :

"SEPIA is given in a routine way for constipation, when there are few symptoms. There is always a sense of fulness in the rectum after stool; ineffectual straining and sweating in the effort because the patient is weak and exhausted. She may go for days with no urging and then the effort is as if she were in labour. Prolapse of the rectum. Weight as of a ball in the anus not relieved by stool. Soreness of the anus. Expulsion of ascarides. Oozing of moisture from the rectum, soreness between buttocks. Haemorrhoids soon form when the rectum is so packed with faeces, and they give additional trouble. With all complaints there is constipation. The bowels lose their ability to expel their contents and the patient is always constipated; constipation during pregnancy; slow, difficult stool, stool like sheep's dung. Always has a feeling of a lump in the rectum never able to empty the bowels; though he goes to stool there is always a sensation of a lump remaining in the rectum. When the stool passes into the lower bowel, it is not expelled until there is an accumulation, which passes the stool out. When these symptoms groups themselves together, the gnawing hunger, the constipation, the dragging down, the mental condition it is SEPIA and SEPIA only."

"The abdomen though distended, has a sensation of emptiness in it. Haemorrhoids are not infrequent. We notice varices in the rectum with great heat and burning and a sensation of heaviness in the anus. The rectum prolapsus particularly after smoking."

Bleeding painful, protruding haemorrhoids, especially with uterine or hepatic disease; soreness, aching or stitches in the anus; when walking ; bleeding when walking.

Dark brown, round balls glued together with mucus.

In the rectum and anus a constricting pain which extends to the perineum or the vagina, sometimes up into the abdomen.

Protrusion of piles and rectum, even after soft stool; worse after drinking milk; continual straining pain in rectum difficulty of urinating, especially in the morning ; a feeling as if drops come out of the bladder, which is not the case; turbid urine of a peculiar foetid odour, depositing, when standing, a lithic acid sediment which adheres tenaciously to the side of the vessel.

Ring of condylomata round anus.

(Weakness of the sphincter; piles come down from any exertion, as walking or standing; she supports the anus by pressure with her hand to prevent protrusion of the parts. The upward stitches in rectum and vagina when present, are equally good indications for SEPIA in cases of haemorrhoids, prolapse of rectum, and for prolapse or induration of uterus

and cervix.)

Silicea :

"The constipation of SILICEA is very remarkable. The stools are extremely hard and large and remaining long in the rectum, as they usually do, they rob the rectum of all its power of expulsion. Though this hard mass of faeces is covered with slime, it takes all his strength to force it to the verge of the anus from which place it unfortunately slips back again. Ultimately he has to remove it mechanically by inserting his finger into his rectum. The straining is violent that even the abdominal walls become sore and the patient breaks out into pools of sweat. Such a constipation, as is to be expected, brings on haemorrhoidal complications. The whole region from anus to rectum becomes intensely painful. Tension at the time of passing stools is so great as to give rise to regular constriction of the anus. The anus also becomes cracked and fissured due to the passage of such enormous lumps of faeces."

After stool, burning in anus; pressure in head; constriction of chest; relief of colic, and great exhaustion; he falls into a slumber from which colic wakes him. Stitching, cutting and burning in rectum and anus. Moisture of the anus.

Haemorrhoidal turmours protrude with stool, return with difficulty, and discharge bloody mucus. Spasmodic, boring, stitching pain from anus up into the rectum and to the testes.

Fissure and fistula ani; also with chest symptoms.

Constipation always before and   during   menses; with irritable sphincter ani.

Inflammation and suppuration of the haemorrhoidal tumours.

Stannum metallicum :

Soreness and smarting at anus, with   fine   stitches, immediately after a stool; itching stitch in rectum.

A corroding pain about anus, while walking and sitting, burning in anus; constant itching.

Violent shooting, like needle pricks at base of rectum extending to anus.

Haemorrhoidal pimple on left side of anus, with painful soreness when touched.

Staphisagria :

Constipation, hard evacuations; tardy without being hard.

Frequent want to evacuate, with scanty evacuations hard or soft. Smarting, sore pain in rectum for long after stool.

Burning cuttings, pressure, and constriction in anus, during evacuation, itching in anus while sitting.

Haemorrhoids, with enlarged prostrate; intense pain in back and through whole pelvis; piles so sensitive that they cannot be touched.

Sulphur :

Constipation; stools hard knotty, insufficient.

SULPHUR constipates, with frequent ineffectual tenesmus, both before and after stool, and constant pressing, even at night, followed by aching and sticking pain in the rectum and anus, often very severe and distressing.

Haemorrhoids; constant ineffectual urging to stool; or thin bloody stool, worse in morning, with soreness of the anus single violent stitches in the rectum, also between stools, arresting the breathing and causing him to start; prolapsus ani during stool, particularly when hard; tensive pain and stiffness in the small of the back, as if the part were too short; inability to stand erect; burning micturition.

He is subject to haemorrhoids, external and internal; great bunches that are sore and raw, burning and tender and that bleed and smart with liquid stool.

After suppression of habitual bleeding; congestion to the head; dizziness; palpitation of the heart; pain in the pit of the stomach, with difficulty of breathing, loss of appetite; sudden hunger faintness before dinner; sleepiness through the day, and sleeplessness at night.

This great antipsoric medicine is often needed at the beginning of a case and may be the only medicine required.

This remedy corresponds to ailments producing haemorrhoids and to troubles resulting from piles which have stopped bleeding, and as a result fulness in the head and uneasiness in the liver.

Sensation in rectum after stool as if something remained.

Bearing down in anus, in forenoon when sitting, with tenesmus.

Anus red, inflamed, swollen, covered with red veins.

Violent stitches and crawling in rectum, especially in evening.

Child afraid on account of pain.

Piles dependent upon abdominal plethora.

Haemorrhoids, blind, or bleeding dark blood, with violent bearing down pain from small of back towards anus.

Painless piles, bleeding, burning and frequent protrusion of the haemorrhoidal tumours; weak digestion, dysuria; shooting in the rectum stops the breathe.

Before stool. Eructation; pinching in abdomen and flatus, causing pain in anus; itching, straining, cutting and sensation like prolapsus in anus; pains in the bladder.

During stool. Burning, sore pain and excoriating cutting in anus; burning, pressing, cutting and prolapse of rectum; piles; cutting in urethra; pains in abdomen and head; accumulation of water in the mouth; nausea, vomiting; catching of breath; palpitation; congestion to the head; chills, particularly about the lower part of body; heat; perspiration.

After stool. Discharge of blood ; sensitiveness, contraction, burning and sensation of soreness and prolapse of anus; straining, jamming, and throbbing in rectum; pressing and stinging in anus and rectum; cramp-like pains in glans and in the ankle of lower jaw; cramp-like twitching about the orifices of the ear; bruised pain and pinching in abdomen; chills and lassitude; thirst.

Sulphuricum acidum :

Stools hard, small black lumps, mixed with blood, with violent pinching in anus ; sediment like blood in the urine; needle-like pains at anus.

Rectum feels as if it had a big ball. Sensation as of rectum being torn asunder during defecation; lancinating pains running upward from anus.

Haemorrhoids feel damp, painful to touch, itch violently; stools cause violent burning, stinging tearing pains of the tumours prevent passage.

Piles burn and fill up the rectum; oozing dampness.

Piles in hard drinkers.

Syphilinum :

The rectum is the seat of many symptoms and conditions.

The constipation of SYPHILINUM is chronic and is of many years' standing ; is due to a kind of stricture high up in the rectum. The rectum feels as if tied up with strictures. The breath of the patient is very foetid.

Ulceration, fissures, nodules, gummata; copious bleeding; cutting burning pains: condylomata.

Paralysis of rectum; prolapsus of anus; relaxed protruding rectum.

Theridion :

Spasmodic contraction of rectum and anus.

Anus protrudes and is painful, aggravated sitting.

Heaviness in the perineal region, which he has had for a very long time, is now felt at every step, with a feeling of a lump there.

Thuja occidentalis :

Constipation, with violent pain, causing stool to recede; stool in hard balls; constipation from inactivity or intrassuception.

Haemorrhoids. During stool, pains are so great she has to desist; burning violently while walking; anus fissured; sensitive to touch; often with warts.

Piles swollen; pain worse sitting, with stitching, burning pains at the anus.

Abrasions of the anus; oozing of fluid from the anus.

Fissures with edges trimmed with polypoid excrescences or true rectal polypus.

Condylomata about the anus, sore to touch; stitches when walking.

Stitches in rectum towards small of back. Pressing, itching and burning in the haemorrhoidal veins.

Offensive perspiration at anus and in perinaeum.

Veratrum album :

Constipation, chronic. Stools : large and hard; or first part large, later parts smaller, stools in round black balls; chronic with children as from inactivity of rectum.

Haemorrhoids, with disease of lungs or pleura.

Painless discharge of masses of blood in clots, with sinking feeling.

Burning sensation in anus, during evacuation; blind piles.

Pressure towards anus ; bruised feeling in sacral region.

Verbascum thapsus :

Haemorrhoids, with obstructed, hardened stool; inflamed and painful piles.

Said to be excellent for itching piles and pruritus ani; one drop of the tincture to the ounce of ointment, applied at bed times.

DR. S.A. JONES gives the following indication as trustworthy:

"Inflamed and very painful piles, scanty evacuation of faeces in small, hard bits, like sheep's dung, with pressing; frequent or copious urination."

Zincum metallicum :

Constipation, stools hard, dry inefficient, only discharged after hard pressing; sensation of soreness and violent itching at anus; tingling at anus as if from worms; violent desire to urinate, worse afternoon, evening, in warm room; better in open air.

Burning in anus during stool.

Feeling in rectum as if flatus pressing against coccyx by which it is retained.

PART II

REPERTORY

Rectum

Abscess : *Calc.*, *cal-s.*, *hep.*, *merc.*, *sil.*, *syph.*, *thuj.*
    just below the coccyx : *Paeon.*
    perineum : *Hep.*, *merc.*, *sil.*

Apthous condition of anus : *Bapt.*, *bor.*, bry., *kali-chl.*, *merc.*, *merc-c.*, *mur-ac.*, *nit-ac.*, *sulph.*, SUL-AC.

Ball in rectum, sensation of : (See Lump.)

Black : Merc-c.

Boils in anus : Cal-p., carb-an., caust., petr.
    near anus : Caust.

Cancer : *Alum.*, *nit-ac.*, ruta, sep.

Catarrh of the rectum (See Mucus, Moisture) *Arg-n.*, aur., *nit-ac.*

Cauliflower exerescence : *Thuj.*

Chilliness in rectum before stool : *Lyc.*

Coldness in anus : All-c., kali-bi., nat-m., sil., sulph.
    afternoon : Kali-bi.
    drops, cold : Cann-s.
    flatus and stool, during : *Con.*
    waking, after : Nat-m., sulph.
    walking in open air, after : Sil.

Condylomata : *Arg-n.*, aur., *aur-m.*, benz-ac., *caust.*, CINNB., *euphr.*, jac-c., lyc., merc., *merc-d.*, *mill.*, *nat-s.*, NIT-AC., petr., phos., sabin., sep., staph., sulph., THUJ.

copious bleeding : *Mill.*
extremely sensitive : STAPH.

flat : *Euphr.*, sulph., THUJ.

sore : Benz-ac., thuj.

Constipation (See Inactivity) : Abies, *abrot.*, AESC., *aeth.*, agar., agn., alet., *aloe*, ALUM., ALUMN., *ambr.*, *am-c.*, *am-m.*, ammc., *anac.*, anan., *ang.*, ant-c., APIS., *arg-m.*, *arg-n.*, arn., ARS., ars-i., arund., asaf., asc-s., asc-t., aster., *aur.*, aur-m., bad., *bar-c.*, *bar-m*, *berb.*, bol., bor., bov., brach., BRY., cact., calad., CALC., *cal-p.*, *cal-s.*, camph., cann-s., *carb-ac.*, carb-an., CARB-S., *carb-v.*, *card-m.*, casc., caul., CAUST., *chel.*, chim., *chin.*, chin-a., chin-s,, cho-ac., cimx., cina., CLEM., *coca*, COCC., COFF., colch., COLL., *coloc.*, CON., *cop.*, cor-r., croc., *crot-c.*, *crot-h.*, crot-t., cub., cupr., cycl., *daph.*, dig., *dios.*, *dulc.*, *elaps.*, ery-a., euon., *ferr.*, *ferr-ar.*, *ferr-i.*, ferr-p., *fl-ac.*, *form.*, *gamb.*, GRAPH., *guaj.*, *hell.*, hep., hippoz., *hydrc.*, *hydr.*, hyos., *hyper.*, *ign.*, *iod.*, *iris.*, jab., jac-c., *jatr.*, *kali-ar.*, *kali-bi.*, *kali-br.*, *kali-c.*, *kali-chl.*, *kali-i.*, kali-p., *kali-s.*, *kreos.*, LACH., LAC-D., *lac-ac.*, *laur.*, led., *lept.*, *lil-t.*, LYC., lycps., mag-c., MAG-M., mag-s., manc., mang., med., meli., *meny.*, *merc.*, merc-c., merc-d., merc-i-f., MEZ., *mosch.*, murx., *mur-ac.*, myric., naja., *nat-a.*, *nat-c.*, NAT-M., nat-p., nat-s., nicc., NIT-AC., *nux-m.*, NUX-V., OENA., olnd., OP., osm., ox-ac., paeon., pall., petr., ph-ac., PHOS., *phyt.*, PLAT., 'PLB., *podo.*, *psor.*, *ptel.*, *puls.*, *pyrog.*, *raph.*, rat., rhus-t., rob.,

Constipation, alternating with diarrhoea.

RUTA., *sabad.*, *sabin.*, sang., SANIC., *sars.*, *sec.*, *seneg.*, SEP., SIL., *spong.*, squil., *stann.*, STAPH., STRAM., STRY., SULPH., *sul-ac.*, sumb., tab., *tarent.*, tell., *ter.*, *ther.*, THUJ., tril., *tub.*, urt-u., ust., vario., *verb.*, VERAT., *vib.*, viol-o., vesp., ZINC.

alternate days, agg. : Alum., *nat-m.*

alternating with diarrhoea : *Abrot.*, acet-ac., agar., ail., aloe., am-m., ANT-C., ant-t., *arg-n.*, *ars.*, ars-i., *aur.*, aur-m-n., berb., *bry.*, *carb-ac.*, carb-s., *card-m.*, *casc.*, CHEL., *cimic.*, cina., *cob.*, coff., *coll.*, *con.*, cop., crot-h., *cupr.*, *dig.*, dios., *ferr-i.*, gamb., graph., grat., *hep.*, ham., *hydr.*, *ign.*, *iod.*, kali-ar., kali-bi., *kali-c.*, kali-s., *lach.*, *lac-d.*, *lact.*, *lec.*, lil-t., *lyc.*, mag-s., *manc.*, *mang.*, merc., mez., nat-a., nat-c., *nat-m.*, nat-p., *nat-s.*, NIT-AC, nux-m., NUX-V., OP., *phos.*, *plb.*, PODO., polyg., *ptel.*, *puls.*, rhus-t., *ruta.*, sang., sars., sep., stram., *sulph.*, sumb., tab., *tub.*, zinc.

aged people, in : ANT-C., bny., nux-v., op., *phos.*

coffee, after : *Mosch.*

constant desire : Aloe., anac., coloc., *con.*, *mag-c.*, mag-m., nat-p., NUX-V., *plb.*, *puls.*, ruta , *sil.*, *sulph.*

difficult stool (See Inactivity) : *Aesc.*, agar., *all-c.*, aloe., ALUM., ALUMN., am-c., AM-M., *anac.*, ANT-C., apis., *aur.*, *aur-m.*, bapt., *bar-c.*, BAR-M., *berb.*, bov., BRY., cact., *calc.*, calc-p., *calc-s.*, *camph.*, canth., CARB-S., *carb-v.*, CAUST., cham., chel., chin., cimx., clem., *cocc.*, colch., coll., coloc., CON., cop., crot-t., dulc., *ferr.*, ferr-i., ferr-p., gels., GRAPH., grat., hell., HEP., *ign.*, *ind.*, iod., kali-bi., *kali-c.*, *kali-p.*, KALI-S., kalm., kreos., LACH., *lac-c.*, LAC-D., lact., laur., *lyc.*, lyss., mag-c., MAG-M., mag-s., mang., meli., *merc.*, merc-c., *mez.*, *mur-ac.*, naja., *nat-c.*, NAT-M., nat-p., nat-s., NIT-AC., NUX-M., NUX-V., Oena., ol-an., olnd., OP., ph-ac., *phos.*, PLAT., PLB., *podo.*, *psor.*, *puls.*, *rat.*, *rhod.*, RUTA., *sabin.*, SANIC., *sars.*, SEL., senec., SEP., SIL., *stann.*, staph., *stram.*, stront., SULPH., sumb., *tarent.*, THUJ., valer., *ver.*, *vib.*, ZINC.

natural stool : Graph., PSOR., SIL.

soft stool : Agn., ALUM., *anac.*, calad., *calc-p.*, *carb-v.*, *chin.*, colch., dulc., gels., graph., *hell.*, HEP., *ign.*, *kali-c.*, *kali-s.*, lach., *lac-c.*, lob., lyc., mag-m., *nat-c.*, *nat-m.*, *nat-s.*, nicc., nit-ac., NUX-M., petr., ph-ac., phos., *psor.*, *puls.*, *rhod.*, *ruta.*, SEP., *sil.*, *stann.*, staph., sulph., tarax., verb., zinc.

stool recedes : Agn., eug., kali-s., *lac-d.*, *mag-m.*, *mur-ac.*, *nat-m.*, OP., sanic., SIL., sulph., thuj.

urinating, can pass stool only when : Aloe, alum.

drugs, after abuse of : Agar., ant-c., *bry.*, chin., COLOC., *hydr.*, lach., NUX-V., *op.*, ruta., sulph.

dryness of rectum, from : *Alum.*
fruitless urging, with (See Ineffectual.)
hard stool, from (See Stool.)
home, when away from : *Lyc.*

Constipation,

    ineffectual urging and straining : Acon., *aesc.*, agar., *all-c.*, aloe., *alum.*, AMBR., ANAC., ant-c., ant-t., arg-m., *arn.*, *ars.*, ars-i., asaf., aster., *bar-c.*, *bell.*, benz-ac., berb., bism., bov., brach., *bry.*, *cact.*, cahin., *calc.*, *calc-s.*, cann-i., cann-s., canth., *caps.*, carb-ac., *carb-an.*, carb-s., *carb-v.*, carl., CAUST., cedr., chel., *chim.*, chin., chin-a., chin-s., cimx., clem., *cocc.*, coc-c., colch., COLL., coloc., CON., corn., crot-t., cupr., cycl., dios., dirc., dros., dulc., elat., eupi., eup-pur., fago., *ferr.*, ferr-ar., ferr-i., ferr-p., fl-ac., form., glon., gran., *graph.*, grat., ham., hell., hep., hura., HYDR., hyper., *ign.*, *iod.*, kali-a., *kali-bi.*, *kali-c.*, kali-n., kali-p., *kali-s.*, *kalm.*, kreos., LACH., *lac-c.*, *lac-d.*, laur., LIL-T., lob-s., LYC., *mag-c.*, MAG-M., mag-s., MERC., merc-c., mosch., myric., nat-a., *nat-c.*, NAT-M., *nat-p.*, nicc., NIT-AC., NUX-V., oena., ol-an., olnd., op., ox-ac., par., petr., phel., ph-ac., *phos.*, phys., phyt., PLAT., plb., podo., psor., ptel., PULS., *rat.*, rheum., rhod., rhus-t., rob., *ruta.*, sabad., sang., *sanic.*, SARS., sec., SEL., SEP., SIL., sol-n., spig., *stann.*, *staph.*, stram., SULPH., sul-ac., sumb., tab., TARENT., tcr., THUJ., til., *verat.*, viol-o., *zinc.*

    evening : *Sil.*

    menses, during : Calc., puls.

  insufficient, incomplete, unstisfactory stools: ALOE., *alum.*, *alumn.*, anac., ang., apis., *arn.*, *bar-c.*, bell., *benz-ac.*, *bry.*, calc., calc-s., carb-ac., carb-s., carb-v., CARD-M.,

> *cham.*, colch., coloc., euphr., *gamb.*, gels., glon., graph.,
> hep., hyos., *ign.*, *iod.*, KLI-C., *kali-s.*, lact., *lyc* ,
> *mag-m.*, mez., naja., NAT-C., NAT-M., NIT-AC.,
> nux-m., NUX-V., oena., OP., par., petr., *plb.*, *pyrog.*,
> rhod., sabad., *sars.*, SEL., seneg., *sep.*, *sil.*, spong.,
> squil., stann., *staph.*, SULPH., *thuj.*, *zinc.*

lean far back to pass a stool, must : *Med.*

menses, before : Am-c., bry., *graph.*, KALI-C., lac-c.,
    lach., mag-c., nat-s., nux-v., SIL., sulph., vesp.

    during: Alum., am-c., am-m., ant-c., APIS., aur., bov.,
        bry., chel., cycl., GRAPH., KALI-C., kali-s., kreos.,
        NAT-M., *nat-s.*, *nux-v.*, phos., PLAT., *plb.*, SEP.,
        SIL., sulph., thuj.

    after : Dirc., graph., lac-c.

    instead of : *Graph.*

    suppressed, during : *Graph.*, ham.

old people : Aloe., alum., alumn., *ant-c.*, *bar-c.*, *bry.*,
    calc-p., *con.*, *lach.*, *nux-v.*, *op.*, *phos.*, *phyt.*, rhus-t.,
    ruta., *sulph.*

painful : Nat-m., NIT-AC., *tub.*

periodic : *Kali-bi.*

    every three weeks : *Kali-bi.*

portal stasis, from : AESC., *aloe.*, NUX-V., SULPH.

pregnancy, during : *Agar.*, alum., *ambr.*, *ant-c.*, *apis.*, *bry.*,
    coll., coloc., *con.*, DOL., *hydr.*, *lyc.*, NAT-S., NUX-V.,
    op., PLB., PLAT., *podo.*, *puls.*, SEP., *sulph.*

seashore, at : Mag-m.

sedantary habits, from : Aloe., *ambr.*, *bry.*, *lyc.*, NUX-V.,
    op., PLAT., *podo.*, *sep.*, *sulph.*

standing, passes stool easier when : CAUST.

stool remains long in the rectum with no urging (See Inactivity) : Am-c., bry., carb-an., cocc., GRAPH., *lach.*, OP., sep.,

with general amel. : Psor.

with awful anxiety : TARENT.

travelling while : *Alum., nux-v., op., plat.*

unable to pass the stool in presence of nurse : AMBR.

vexation, after : Bry., nux-v., staph.

wine, after : *zinc.*

CONSTRICTION, contraction, closure, etc, : Acon., *aesc.,* aeth., *agar.,* alum., am-c., arg-n., ars., *bell.,* benz-ac., berb., bor., *cact., calc.,* cal-s , *camph., cann-s.,* carb-an., carb-v., CAUST., *chel.,* chin., cic., cimx., *cocc.,* coff., *colch.,* coloc., cop.. crot-t., der., ferr. ferr-ar., ferr-i., ferr-p., *fl-ac.,* form., graph., grat., guarc., hipp., hura., *hyos.,* IGN., kali-ar., *kali-bi., kali-br.,* kali-c., LACH., laur., LYC., marg., meli., mez., nat-c., *nat-m.,* nat-p., NIT-AC., NUX-V., *op., phos.,* PLB., rat., *rhus-t.,* sars., sec., *sep.,* sil., sol-t., staph., stront., *sulph.,* sumb., syph., *tab.,* ther., thuj., verb.

morning : Nux-v.

rising, after : Nux-v.

forenoon : *Calc.*

afternoon : *cocc.,* coloc.

evening : *Ign.*

walking, while : Ign.

night : Sec.

alternating with itching : *Chel.*

Constriction

    breakfast, after : calc-s.

    coition, during : Merc-c.

    flatus, passing : Fl-ac.

    lying amel. : *Mang.*

    menses, during : *Cocc.*, thuj.

    mental exertion, after : Nux-v.

    motion amel : Coloc.

    painful : Brach., *calc.*, *caust.*, *cocc.*, coloc., IGN., LACH., *lyc.*, *mang.*, *mez.*, NUX-V., PLB., *sep.*, *sil.*, thuj.

    prolapsed anus : *Lach.*, *mez.*

    sitting, while : *Cocc.*, *mang.*

        amel : *Ign.*

        rising from : Thuj.

    spasmodic : Chel., coff., grat., *ham* , *hipp.*, *lach.*, *lyc.*, merc-*c.*, nat-m., NIT-AC., NUX-V., OP., *phos.*, PLB., verb.

    standing agg. : *Ign.*

    stool, before : *Ham.*, *lach.*, nat-m., *nux-v.*, phos., plb., sep.

        during : *Alum.*, *ars.*, *chel.*, chin-s., coloc., ferr., glon., *kreos.*, mang., NAT-M., NIT-AC., nux-m., *nux-v.*, phos., PLB., sep., SIL., *thuj.*

        after : Aesc., chel , colch., elaps., *ferr.*, form., grat., IGN., kali-bi., LACH., *mez.*, NIT-AC., nux-m., *phos.*, plat., *sep.*, stront., *sulph.*, thuj.

        preventing : All-c., *berb.*, *chel.*, *lach.*, LYC., *nat-m.*, nit-ac., *nux-v.*

        urging to, during : Caust.

    urinating, on : Carb-s., nat-m.

        at close of : *Cann-s.*

walking, on : *Caust*., crot-t.

extending into rectum : Sil.

upward : Laur., sil.

testes, to : Chin., sil.

vagina, to : Sep.

Cramp. (See Constriction.)

Perineum : Sulph., thuj.

Crawling in (See Formication, Itching.)

Difficult stool (See Constipation.)

Distension : Agar., op.

Dragging, heaviness, weight : Acon., AESC., agar., ALOE, ang., ant-c., arn., bar-c., bell., berb., bry., *cact*., calc., cann-s., *carb-v*., caust., chel., coll., con., crot-t., cycl., euphr., graph., hep., hyos., inul., kali-bi., kali-c., kali-n., kali-p., kreos., lach., lact., laur., led., lil-t., lob., lyc., mag-m., manc., merc., *nit-ac*., nux-m., nux-v., phos., plan., plb., puls., rhus-t., sacc., sep., staph , sulph., sumb., ther., thuj., verat., *zinc*.

morning : Lyc.

stool, after : Lyc.

afternoon : Cycl.

dinner, after : Cycl.

sleep, after : Cycl.

evening, during loose stool : Op.

menses, before : Phos.

during : *Aloe*.

standing, while : *Zinc*.

Dragging

> stool, before : Hell., merc.
>> during : Mez., *nit-ac.*, op.
>> after : Hell., kali-bi., nat-m., rhus-t., ruta., zinc.
>> amel., after : kreos.
> Perineum : Cann-s., graph., nat-a., puls., ther.

Draw in, desire to, anus : Agar.

Dryness : AESC.,   aeth.,   agar.,   *alumn.*,   calc.,   carb-v.,
> graph., *kali-chl.*, *nat-m.*, sulph., sumb.
> sensation of : Agar., calc., carb-v.

Eruption about anus : *Agar.*, am-c., am-m., ant-c., ars., berb.,
> *calc.*, carb-an., carb-s., carb-v., *caust.*, *graph.*, hep., ign.,
> kali-c., lyc., med., merc., NAT-M., nat-s., NIT-AC.,
> PETR.,   sep., *staph.*, *sulph.*, thuj.

> blotches : Carb-v., stann., *staph.*, *thuj.*
> burning : Ars., calc.
> crust : Berb.
> herpectic : *Berb.*, *graph.*, lyc., *nat-m.*, PETR.
> itching : Ars., cinnb., lyc., PETR., staph., sulph.

> pimples : Agar., brom., carb-v., cinnb., kali-c., kali-i.,
>> nit-ac., staph.

> pustules : Amm-m., calc., caust.
> scurfy : *Petr.*
> stinging : Nit-ac.
> ulcerous : Kali-c.
> vesicular : Brom., carb-v.
> warmth of bed agg. : *Petr.*

Perineum : Brom., graph., *petr.*, sars., *sulph.*, tell., tep.

    boil : Ant-c.

    dry : *Petr.*

    herpes : Kali-c., PETR., tell.

    pimples : Nit-ac., sep., sulph., sul-ac.

Excoriation : *Aesc., agar.,* agn., all-c., alum., am-c., *apis.,* arg-m., *ars.,* asc-c., aur-m., *bar-c., berb., calc.,* calc-s., carb-an., CARB-S., CARB-V., CAUST., *cham.,* coloc., ferr., *gamb.,* GRAPH., grat., hep., *hydr., ign.,* kali-ar., kali-c., lach., LYC., *merc.,* merc-c., mur-ac , nat-a., *nat-m.,* nat-p., *nit-ac.,* nux-v., *petr.,* phos., plant., *podo., puls., sanic., sep.,* SULPH., sumb., *syph.,* thuj., tub., urt-u., zinc.

acrid moisture, from : Carb-v., *merc-c.,* *thuj.,* zinc.

riding on horseback : Carb-an.

    in a wagon : Psor.

must rub anus until raw : *Agar.,* alum., am-c., *arg-n., bar-c., calc.,* carb-s., CARB-V., CAUST., GRAPH., kali-c., LYC., *merc.,* PETR., phos., *puls., sep.,* SULPH.

stools, from the : ALOE, APIS, *ars., bapt.,* coloc., *kreos., merc.,* mur-a., NIT-AC., nux-m., *nux-v.,* rheum., sang., *sulph., tub.*

Nates, between : Arg-m., arum-t., *berb.,* calc., *carb-s.,* carb-v., *graph., kreos.,* nat-m., *nit-ac.,* puls., *sep., sulph.*

    walking, from : Ang-m., CAUST., nat-m., *nit-ac.*

Perineum, of : Alum., arum-t., aur-m., *calc.,* carb-an., *carb-v., caust., cham., graph., hep.,* ign., LYC., *merc.,* petr., puls., rhod., sep., *sulph.,* thuj.

Feces remained in, as if : *Graph. lyc.*, NAT-M., nit-ac., SEP., verat.

Fissure : Aesc., *agn.*, all-c., alum., ant-c., arg-m., *ars.*, arum t., berb., calc., calc-fl., *calc-p.*, carb-an., caust., CHAM., *cund.*, cur., *fl-ac.*, GRAPH., grat., hydr., *ign.*, kali-c., *lach.*, med., *merc.*, merc-i-r., mez., mur-ac., *nat-m.*, NIT-AC., *nux-v.*, *paeon.*, *petr.*, *phos.*, *phyt.*, plat., *plb.*, RAT., rhus-t., SEP., *sil.*, *sulph.*, syph., THUJ.

Fistula : *Aloe.*, *alum.*, ant-c., aur., AUR-M., bell., BERB., bry., cact., CALC., CALC-P., calc-s., carb-s., CARB-V., CAUST., *fl-ac.*, *graph.*, hep., *hydr.*, ign., KALI-C., *kreos.*, *lach.*, *lyc.*, *merc.*, NIT-AC., *petr.*, *phos.*, puls., *sep.*, SIL., *staph.*, *syph.*, thuj.,

pulsating : *Caust.*

Foreign body, sensation of : Lil-t, nat-m., rumx., sep., sulph.

Formication in anus : *Aesc.*, agar., ail., aloe, all-c., alum., ambr., ant-c., ant-t., arg-m., arg-n., *bar-c.*, benz-ac., berb., bov., CALC., CALC-S., canth., carb-s., *carb-v.*, caust., chel., chin., *cinnb.*, COC-C., colch., croc., elaps., fago., ferr-i., ferr-ma., gran., grat., hep., *ign.*, KALI-C., kali-p., kreos., mez., mosch., *mur-ac.*, *nat-c.*, *nux-v.*, ol-an., phos., *plat.*, plb., rhod., rhus-t., *sabad.*, *sep.*, sil., spig., spong., SULPH., ter., *teucr.*, verat-v., *zinc.*

evening : Euphr., plat., spong., *sulph.*, teucr.

in bed : Plat., *teucr.*

night : *Nux-v.*

sitting, while : SULPH.
stool, before : Phos.
after : Aloe., berb., mez., teucr.
Perineum : Acon., chel., petros., rhod.

Fulness : Acon., AESC., agar., ALOE., alum., apis., ars., bell., berb., bry., carb-v,, caust., cycl., ferr., HAM., kali-bi., *lach.*, lil-t., manc., med., meli., NIT-AC., phos., plan., sabin., stram., SULPH., thuj.

alternating with sensation of emptiness : Thuj.
stool, after : AESC., alum., *lyc.*, *sep.*
walking, after : Aesc.
Perineum : Alum., berb., bry., *chin.*, cycl., nux-v.

Grumbling: Mang.

Gurgling in rectum : Calc., carb-an., laur., stry., *sulph.*

Haemorrhage from anus : Acet-ac., ACON., *aesc.*, agar., aloe., alum., *alumn.*, ambr., *am-c.*, am-m., anac., aur., aur-m., bapt., BAR-C., bar-m., *bell.*, berb,, *bism.*, *bor.*, bufo., CACT., CALC., calc-fl., *calc p*, *calc-s.*, camph., *canth.*, *caps.*, carb-an., *carb-s.*, *carb-v.*, card-m., carl., CASC., *cham.*, *chin.*, chin-a., chin-s., chlor., chrom-ac., cob., *cocc.*, COLL., coloc., CROT-H., cycl., dios., elaps., *erig.*, *eug.*, *ferr.*, ferr-ars., ferr-m., ferr-p., ficcus., *fl-ac.*, *graph.*, HAM., *hep.*, hydr., *hyos.*, hyper., *ign.*, *ip.*, *kali-ar.*, *kali-bi.*, kali-c,- *kali-chl.*, *kali-i.*, kali-m., kali-n., kali-p., kali-s., LACH., led., *lept.*, lob.,

Haemorrhage

       LYC., lyss., manc., med., *merc.*, *merc-c.*, *mill.*, *mur-ac.*,
       NAT-M., *nat-s.*, NIT-AC., nux-m., NUX-V., operc.,
       paeon., ph-ac., PHOS., *phyt.*, plat., *podo.*, PSOR., *puls.*,
       pyrog., *rat.*, rhus-t., rhus-v., *ruta.*, sabin., scrouph., *sep.*,
       sil., stram., SULPH., thalapsi., thuj., valer., varat., zinc.

morning : Plan.

       stool, after : Puls.

afternoon : Sulph.

evening, stool, during : Calc.

night : NIT-AC.

black : Aloe, alumn., ant-c., colch., crot-h., *ham.*, hydr.,
       kali-m., merc-c., *sec.*, sulph.

       liquid : Elaps.

exertion after : Berb.

flatus, during emission of : Phos.

menses, before : Am-c.

       during ; Am-m ; ars-m., *graph.*, LACH., lyss.

       scanty, during : LACH.

       suppressed : Graph., ham., zinc.

periodic : Mur-ac., nit-ac.

rubbing, on : Aesc.

stool, during : *Alum.*, alumn., *ambr.*, Am-c., am-m., aur.,
       aur-m., bufo., *calc-p.*, *carb-an.*, *carb-v.*, HAM., *hep.*,
       ign., *kali-c.*, lyc., NAT-M., *nit-ac.*, nux-v., plan.,
       PHOS., *puls.*, rheum., tub.

       after: *Agar.*, aloe., *alum.*, Am-c., *calc-p.*, carb-s., *carb-v.*,
       chel., cycl., fl-ac., grat., *ign.*, *kali-c.*, kali-n., *lach.*,
       merc., mez., nat-m., *phos.*, rhus v., sel., sep.,
       spong., sulph.

from hard : *Fl-ac.*, *kali-c.*, NAT-M., prun., tub.
walking, while : Alum., sep.

Haemorrhoids : Abrot., acet-ac., acon., aesc-gl., AESC., aeth., AGAR., agn., ALOE, alum., alumn., ambr., *am-c.*, am-m., anac., anan., ang., *ant-c.*, ant-t., *apis.*, apoc., arg-n., arn., ARS., ars-i., arum-t., aur., aur-m., bapt., *bar-c.*, *bell.*, berb., bor., bov.; *brom.*, bry., *bufo.*, cact., *calc.*, calc-fl., *calc-p.*, *calc-s.*, cann-s., *canth.*, carb-ac., CARB-AN., CARB-V., carb-s., *card-m.*, carl., casc., CAUST., cham., *chel.*, chim., chin., chin-a., chr-ac., cic., cimic., *cimx.*, clem., coca., cocc., *coff.*, colch., COLL., *coloc.*, con., cop., croc., crot-h., cycl., *dios.*, elaps., *erig.*, *eug.*, euphr., *ferr.*, *ferr-ar.*, ferr-m., ferr-p., *fl-ac.*, gels.. GRAPH., grat., HAM., *hell.*, hep., *hydr.*, hyos., hyp , *ign.*, iod., *ip.*, KALI-AR., *kali-bi.*, KALI-C., kali-n kali-p., KALI-S., kreos., LACH., lact., *lept.*, lil-t., lob., LYC., mag-m., manc., med., *merc.*, MERC-I-R., mez., mill., mosch., mucuna., MUR-AC., *nat-m.*, nat-s., negundo., NIT-AC., NUX-V., PAEON., *petr.*, ph-a., PHOS., phy., phyt., pinus-sylv., plan., plat., plb., *podo.*, polyg., *psor.*, PULS., Radium., *rat.*, *rhus-t.*, rhus-v., rumx., ruta., *sabin.*, *sang.*, scrophul., sec., sedum., semper-t., SEP., *sil.*, stann., staph., stront., SULPH., *sul-ac* , sumb., syph., *ter.*, ther., *thuj.*, tub., verat., verat-v., wythe., zinc., *zing.*
    aggravation, confinement, after : Aloe, apis.
    stool after, for hours : *Aesc.*, Amm-m., ign., rat., sul.
    as rheumatic symptoms abate : Abrot.
    climacteric, during : Aesc., lach.

Haemorrhoids (CONTD.)

       sitting, during : Graph., ign., *thuj.*

       abuse of alcoholic drinks in sedentary persons :
          Aesc-gl., nux-v.

       coughing, sneezing, from : Caust., *kali-c.*, lach.

       leucorrhoea, suppressed : Am-m.

       talking, thinking of them, from : Caust.

       walking, from : Caust, sep.

amelioration, cold water, from : *Aloe.*, nux-v., rat.

       hot water from : *Ars.*, mur-ac.

       lying down, from : Am-c.

       walking, from : Ign.

morning agg. : Aloe., DIOS., mur-ac , sabin., sulph., sumb.,
       thuj.

       amel : Alum., coll.

       bed, in, agg. : Graph., rumx.

       waking him : Aloe., kali-bi., petr., sulph.

night agg. : Aesc., aloe., alum., am-c., ant-c., ars., carb-an.,
       carb-v., coll., euphr., ferr., graph., *merc.*, phys., *puls.*,
       rhus-t., SULPH.

alternating with palpitation : COLL.

       with lumbago : *Aloe.*

backache, with : Aesc-gl., *Aesc.*, *bell.*, calc-fl., chrom-ac.,
       euonym., ham., *ign.*, nux-v., sulph.

beer agg. : Aloe., bry., ferr., nux-v., rhus-t., SULPH.

bleeding : (See Haemorrhage from anus).

blind : AESC., ant-c., ars, brom., caps., calc-fl., *calc-p.*,
       cham., *coll.*, ferr., grat., *ign.*, mucuna., nit-ac.,
       nux-v., podo., *puls.*, *rhus-t.*, *sulph.*, wythe., verat.

Haemorrhoids :

bluish : Aesc-gl., AESC., aeth., aloe., ars., caps., CARB-V., dios., *ham.*, LACH., *lyc.*, manc., MUR-AC., phys., *sulph.*, verat-v.

children, in : *Mur-ac.*

chronic : AESC., *aloe.*, am-c., calc., carb-v., *carb-s.*, caust., COLL., dios., graph., *lach.*, *lyc.*, MERC-I-R., *nit-ac.*, NUX-V., petr., *phos.*, phyt., *podo.*, SULPH., *tub.*

cold amel. : Aloe., brom.

colic, haemorrhoidal : Carb-v., coloe., lach., *nux-v.*, puls., *sulph.*

congested : *Acon.*, agar., *aloe.*, alum., apoc., arg-n., ars., *bell.*, carb-v., *caust.*, *cham.*, *hep.*, KALI-C., kali-n., *merc.*, *mur-ac.*, NUX-V., PAEON., podo., *puls.*, *rhus-t.*, sil., *sulph.*, verat-v., zinc.

disposition, haemorrhoidal : Aesc., calc., carb-v., caust., graph., lach., nux-v., petr., sulph.

delility, with : Ars., cinch., ham., hydr., mur-ac.

drunkards, in : *Ars.*, *carb-v.*, NUX-V., *sul-ac.*

epistaxis, with : Carb-v.

excitement : Arg-n., gels., hyos., nat-c., nux-v., sumb.

external : Abrot., AESC., all-c.. ALOE., alum., *am-c.*, anac., *ang.*, ant-c., apis., apoc., arn., ars., ars-i., aur., *bar-c.*, bar-m., berb., *brom.*, bry., cact., *calc.*, *cal-p.*, cal-s., caps., carb-ac., carb-an., *carb-s.*, carb-v., *caust.*, *coll.*, coloc., dios., *ferr.*, *ferr-ar.*, ferr-i., ferr-p., fl-ac., *gran.*, *graph* , grat., HAM., *hep.*, *iod..* kali-ar., kali-c., kali-n., kali-p., kali-s., LACH., *lyc.*, med., *merc.*, MUR-AC., nat-m., *nit-ac.*, nux-v., *paeon.*, ph-ac., *phos.*, phys., *plat.*, *podo*, *puls*, RAT., rumx., *rhus-t.*,

Haemorrhoids (CONTD.) :

sep., *sil.*, SULPH., sul-ac., *ter.*, thuj., *tub.*, verat., zinc.

flatus, protrude when passing : *Bar-c., phos.*

hard : Ail., alum., ambr., CAUST., *lach., lyc.,* phys., *sep.*

heart disease, with : Cact., coll., dig.

hypochondriasis, with : Aesc., grat., *nux-v.*

inflamed (See Congested).

infants, of : Am-c., bor., coll., merc.

internal : *Aesc., alum.,* ant-c., arn., ARS., bor., BROM., *calc., caps.,* caust., CHAM., cimic., COLOC., hep., IGN., kali-ar., kali-c., kali-p., kali-s., *lach.,* lyc., NUX-V., *petr., ph-ac.,* phos., *plant.,* PODO., PULS., *rhus-t.,* sep., stront., SULPH., *ter.,* verat.

irreducible : Ars., atrop., sil., sulph.

itching : (See Itching).

large : AESC., agar., ALOE., alum., ang., arn., ars., bry., *cact., calc.,* caps., CARB-AN., *carb-s., carb-v.,* CAUST., clem., *coloc.,* cycl., *dios.,* euphr., ferr., ferr-ar., gal-ac., *graph.,* HAM., kali-ar., KALI-C., kali-n., kali-s., *lach.,* lyc., manc., *merc., mur-ac.,* nat-m., NIT-AC., NUX-V., *podo., puls.,* sep., SULPH., sulp-ac., thuj., *tub.*

menses, before : Cocc., phos., puls.

during, agg. : *Aloe.,* am-c., calc.. *carb-s., carb-v.,* cocc., *coll., graph., ign., lach.,* lyss., phos., *puls.,* sulph.

after, agg. : Cocc.

Haemorrhoids (CONTD.) :

    suppressed, during : Phos., *sulph.*

mental exertion : *Caust.*, nat-c.

mercury, after abuse of : *Hep.*, sul-ac.

milk agg. : *Sep.*

motion agg. : Apis, carb-an., euphr., merc., *mur-ac.*, nat-m., puls.

mucous : Aesc., Ant-c., bor., caps., *carb-v.*, graph., ign., lach., merc., nux-v., *phos.*, *puls.*, Ran-b., *Sulph.*

muco-bloody discharge, with : Ant-c., bor., ign., merc., puls.

muco-purulent : Ant-c., hep., lyc.

offensive (fetid) : Carb-v., manc., med.

old people, of : Am-c., anac.

parturition agg. : *Ign.*, KALI-C., lil-t., *mur-ac.*, *podo.*. *puls.*, sep., *sulph.*

pendulus : Nit-ac.

plethora, abdominal, with : *Aesc.*, *aloe.*, coll., ham., negundo, nux-v., sep., sulph.

pregnancy, during : *Aesc.*, *am-m.*, ant-c., *caps.*, *coll.*, *lach.*, *lyc.*, *nat-m.*, *nux-v.*, sep., *sulph.*

protruding, but easily replaced : Ign.

purgatives, after : Aloe., *nux-v.*

rheumatism abates, after : Abrot.

round the anus, like a pad : Aesc., aloe., calc., coll., mur-ac., nux-v.

riding amel. : *Kali-c.*

standing agg. : *Aesc.*, *am-c.*, *caust.*, *sulph.*

Haemorrhoids (CONTD.) :

    stool, preventing : *Aesc., caust., lach., paeon.,* sul-ac., *thuj.,*

        protrude during: Alumn., *am-c., bar-c., calc.,* CALC-P.,
            fl-ac., kali-bi., *kali-c.,* lach., *mur-ac., nit-ac.,* phos.,
            ph-ac., plat., RAT., *rhus-t., sil.*

        grape-like, swollen : *Aesc., aloe., am-c.,* caps., carb-v.,
            caust., coll., diosc., graph., ham., kali-c., lach.,
            mur-ac., nux-m., *nux-v.,* rat., scrophul., sep.,
            sulph., thuj.

        when urinating : Bar-c., mur-ac.

    strangulated : *Aesc.,* ALOE., ars., *bell., ign.,* LACH., lob.,
        nux-v., PAEON., sep., *sil., sulph.*

    suppressed : Ars., *calc.,* caps., carb-v., euphr., NUX-V.,
        phos, puls., SULPH.

    suppurating : Anan., *carb-v., hep., ign.,* merc., SIL.

    thinking of them agg. : *Caust.*

    touch agg. : Abrot., BELL., berb., calc., carb-an., carb-s.,
        CAUST., graph., *hep., kali-c.,* lit-t., lyc., merc.,
        MUR-AC., nit-ac., nux-v., phos., RAT., sep., sil.,
        SULPH., sul-ac., syph., THUJ.

    ulcerating : *Cham., hep., ign.,* kali-c., *lach.,* nit-ac., *paeon.,*
        phos., SIL., staph., syph.

    urination, protrude during : Aloe., BAR-C., *bar-m.,*
        canth., kali-c., merc., *mur-ac.,* nit-ac.

        after, agg. : Merc.

    walking agg. : AESC., agn., alum., ars., brom., calc.,
        CARB-AN., CAUST., cycl., kali-ar., kali-c.,
        MUR-AC., nit-ac., phos., phys., rumx., sep., sil.,
        SULPH., sumb., ther., thuj.

Haemorrhoids (CONTD.) :
  walkins. amel : IGN.
  warmth, external., amel. : *Ars.*, *mur-ac.*
    warm weather agg. : Nit-ac.
    amel. : *Aesc.*

  wiping after stool agg. : AESC., GRAPH., MUR-AC., PAEON., puls., *sulph.*
Heaviness (See Dragging.)

Itching : Acon., AESC., AGAR., agn., *all-c.*, ALOE., *alum.*, alumn., *ambr.*, AM-C., *am-m.*, anac., *ant-c.*, apis., apoc., arg-m., *arg-n.*, ars., ars-i., aur-s., bar-c., bar-m., *bell.*, *berb.*, bor., bov., brom., bry., bufo., cact., cahin., CALC., *calc-ar.*, *calc-p.*, CALC-S., *caps*, carb-ac., CARB-S., CARB-V., card-m., *carl.*, CAUST., cham., *chel.*, chin., chin-a., chin-s., *cic.*, *cina.*, cinnb., cist., *clem.*, cocc., coc-c., coff., *colch.*, *coll.*, coloc., con., *croc.*, crot-t., dios., *dulc.*, elaps., *euph.*, ferr., ferr-ar., ferr-ma., ferr-m., ferr-p., FL-AC., GRAPH., *gran.*, grat., *ham.*, hep., hydc., *ign.*, *iod.*, *ip.*, jac-c., jug-r., *kali-ar.*, kali-bi., KALI-C., kili-n., kali-p., KALI-S., *lach.*, led., lil-t., lith., LYC., mag-c., mag-m., med., *merc.*, *mez.*, *mill.*, morph., *mur-ac.*, naja., *nat-a.*, NAT-C., *nat-m.*, *nat-p.*, nat-s., NIT-AC., NUX-V., op., ox-ac., *paeon.*, *petr.*, phel., ph-ac., PHOS., *plat.*, plb., prun., psor., PULS., ran-s., *rat.*, rhus-t., *rhus-v.*, *rumx.*, *ruta.*, *sabad.*, sabin., *sars.*, sec., *sep.*, serp., *sil.*, sin-a., *spig.*, *spong.*, squil., *stann.*, *staph.*, SULPH., *sul-ac.*, *sul-i.*, syph., tab., *teucr.*, thuj., *tub.*, urt-u., wye., *zinc.*, zing.

Itching (CONTD.) :

   daytime : SULPH.

   morning : Agar., carb-v., carb-s., cench., jac-c., lach., nat-m., *sulph*.

      bed, in : Carb-v.

   forenoon : Dios , peaon.

   evening : Alumn., bor., *calc-p*, cham., croc, *iod.*, kali-bi., lyc., nux-v., phos., *plat.*, *puls.*, ran-s., sil , *sulph.*, thuj., zinc.

      bed, in : Ant-c., cahin., calc-p., cinnb., *ign.*, *lyc* ., nat-m., petr , plat , *sulph.*, *teucr*.

   night : Agar , aloe., alum., alumn., ant-c., calc-f., carb-s , *ferr* , fl-ac., *ign.*, *nat-p.*, petr., phos., rhus-v., *sulph.*,

      midnight, before : Thuj.

   alternating with ear : Sabad.

   ascarides, from : *Calc.*, calc-f., chin., ferr., ign., *nat-p.*, *sabad.*, sin-a., *teucr.*, *urt-u.*

   burning : *Agar* , *alumn* , ant-c., *berb.*, bufo., calc., carb-s., chin., cocc., *iod.*, jug-r., kali-c., lyc., mur-ac., paeon., rhus-v., sars., SULPH., *thuj*.

   coition, after : Anac.

   cold bathing amel. : Aloe., caust., fl-ac.

   dinner, after : Caust.

   discharge of moisture, after : *Sulph*.

   menses, during : carb-v.

   pain, ending in : *Zinc*.

   riding, while : Bov.,

   rubbing agg. : *Alum.*, petr.

Itching (CONTD.) :

scratching agg. : *Agar.*, *alum.*, arg-m., ars., bar-c., calc., *caps.*, carb-v., *caust.*, chel., con., merc., *mez.*, mur-ac., nat-c., petr. : pho-ac., phos., *puls.*, rhus-t., rhus-v., sep., *sil.*, stann., *staph.*, SULPH.

sitting, while : Jac-c., *staph.*

sleep, on going to : Petr.
    after : *Lach.*

stool, before : Euph., *spong.*
    during : Kali-c., merc., mur-ac., nat-m., phos., pic-ac., sil., *sulph.*, teucr.

    after : Agar., aloe., alum., berb., bov., cahin., calc.. carb-s., carb-v., clem., *euph.*, eupi., *kali-c.*, lyc., mag-m., ʻmerc., *mur-ac.*, *nat-m.*, nicc., nit-ac., pic-ac., plat., ptel., sec., *sil.*, *staph.*, sulp., tell., ter., teucr., thuj., zinc.

    amel. : Clem.
stooping, on : Arg-m.

voluptuous : *Agar.*, *alum.*, ambr., arg-m., *carb-v.*, cina., merc., mur-ac., petr., plat., *puls.*, sep., *sil.*, spig., SULPH.

walking., while : Aesc., kali-bi., nat-m., nit-ac., nux-v., phos.

    in open air : Arg-m., nit-ac.

warm bed, in : *Alum.*, cahin., calc-p., carb-v., *ign.*, *lvc.*, *nat-p.*, *petr.*, *suph.*, *teucr.*

Itching (CONTD.) :

    extending into urethra during stool : Thuj.

        around anus : Agn., *berb.*, bry., buf-s., *fl-ac.*, lyc., *mez.*, nat-s., *nux-v.*, op., PETR., serp., SULPH., tarax.

    warmth of bed : *Petr.*

    Perineum : Ang., *alum.*, ars., bell., canth., cann-s., carb-v., *chel.*, cina., con., *fl-ac.*, gran., ign., kali-c., mur-ac., nat-c., *nat-s.*, nux-v., PETR., plb., *sars.*, seneg., SULPH., tep., thuj.

    forenoon : Thuj.

    night : *carb-v.*, kali-c., petr.

    scratching agg. : Alum.

        after, pain : Alum.

    stool, during : *Sulph.*

    touched, when : *Carb-v.*

    walking, while : Ign.

Lump, sensation of (See Weight) : Aloe., anac., apoc., bry., cann-i., *caust.*, *crot-t.*, *kali-bi.*, *lach.*, lit-t., med., *nat-m.*, rumx., sacc., sang., sarr., SEP,, *sil.*, sulph., ther.

    menses, during : *Sil.*

    sitting agg. : Cann-i., kali-bi., lach., nat-m.

    standing agg. : *Lil-t.*

    stool, not amel. by : SEP.

        before : *Lach.*

    Perineum : CHIN., *ther.*

Moisture : Acon., *aesc.*, agar., *aloe.*, *alum.*, am-c., anac., ANT-C., apis., ars., aur., bapt., *bar-c.*, *bar-m.*, bell., *bor.*, bry., *calc.*, cal-p., *cal-s.*, *canth.*, caps., *carb-an.*,

Moisture (CONTD.) :

> CARB-S., CARB-V., carl., CAUST., chel., chin.,
> chin-a., clem., coc-c., coff., *colch.*, coloc., cor-r., *dios.*,
> dulc., ferr., ferr-ar., ferr-p., GRAPH., *hell.*, HEP., ign.,
> *lach.*, led., lyc., med., meli., *merc.*, *merc-c.*, mill.,
> *mur-ac.*, nat-m., NIT-AC., *nux-v.*, *paeon.*, *petr.*, *phos.*,
> *phyt.*, podo., *puls* , ran-s., *rat.*, rhus-t., SEP., SIL., spig.,
> stann., SUPLH., sul-ac., syph.; *thuj* , zinc.

evening : Carb-an., dios.

night : *Carb-v.*, nat-m.

acrid : Carb-v., *merc-c.*, *nit-ac.*, *thuj.*, zinc.

bloody : Alum., *carl.*, sabad., *sil* , thuj.

flatus, from : All-c., *ant-c.*, *carb-v.*, zinc.

glutinous : *Carb-v.*, GRAPH.

herring brine, smelling like : *Calc.*, *med.*

menses, during : LACH.

musty odor : *Carb-v.*

scratching : *Alum.*, CARB-V., dulc., GRAPH., *lyc.*, *merc.*,
> *nat-m.*, *nit-ac.*, *petr.*, rhus-t., *sep.*, sil., SULPH., sul-ac.,
> *thuj.*

stool, before : Kali-c.
> after : Bor., *graph.*, *sep.*, stann., sumb., zinc.

Perineum : Carb-an., *carb-v.*
> night : *Carb-v.*

Numbness of anus : Acon., carb-a., phos.

Open anus (See Relaxed) : Aesc., *phos.*, *sec.*, sol-t-ae.

sensation of : Aloe., *apis.*, apoc., *phos.*, puls., sumb.

> stool, after : Apoc., sumb.

Pain : Acon., AESC., agar., all-c., *aloe.*, *alum.*, *alumn.*, AM-C., am-m., anac., ant-c., arn., *ars.*, ars-i., bar-c., bar-m., bell., berb., BROM., bry., *bufo.*, cact., calad., calc., cal-p., calc-s., camph., canth., caps., *carb-an.*, *carb-s:*, *carb-v.*, carl., CAUST., cham., chel , chin., chin-a., chr-ac., cimic., cocc., colch., COLL., *coloc.*, con., croc., cupr., cycl., dios., dulc., euphr., ferr., ferr-ar., ferr-p., GRAPH., grat., ham., hell., IGN., iod., iris., *kali-ar.*, kali-bi., KALI-C., kali-chl., kali-n., kali-p., kali-s., lac-ac., lach., *lil-t.*, LYC , mag-c., med., *merc.*, mez., mill., *mur-ac.*, nat-c., nat-m., nat-p., *nit-ac.*, *nux-v* , PAEON., phel., ph-ac., *phos.*, phys., phyt., plb., *podo.*, *psor.*, PULS., *rat.*, rhus-t., rhus-v., rumx., *ruta.*, sabad., sars., sec., seneg., *sep.*, sil., stann., stornt., SULPH., sul-ac., sumb., syph., tarent., ther., THUJ., valer., zinc., zing.

 morning : Calc-p., dios., *kali-bi.*, podo.

  stool, during : *podo.*

  after : *Kali-bi.*

  7 a.m : Nat-m.

 forenoon : Kali-bi., nat-m., thuj.

  10 a.m. sitting while : SEP.

 afternoon : Chel., *cocc.*, cycl.

 evening : Carb-v., dios., *lach.*, mez., nux-v., *sulph.*

  lying, while : *Ign.*

 night : Mosch., ox-ac., *puls.*

  midnight : Nux-v.

4 a.m. : *Mag-c.*

coition, after : Caust.

Pain (CONTD.) :

continuous : Am-c., am-m., calc., graph., ign., kali-c.,
lyc., *nit-ac.*, nux-v., sep., stront.

convulsive : *Lach.*, lyc., psor., sang.

cough, from : *Kali-c.*, *lach.*

eating, after : Lyc., nux-v.

flatus, on passing : Camph., carb-v.

kneeling amel. : *Aesc.*

lying agg. : *Aesc.*, crot-t., phos., *puls.*

on abdomen, amel : Nux-v.

back : Chel.

amel : Alumn., *am-c.*, mang.

menses, before : Ign., petr.

during : *Aloe.*, ars., berb., phos.

mental exertion, after : *Caust.*, nux-v.

motion agg. : *Nux-v.*, *thuj.*

periodical, everyday : *Ign.*

pressing upon umblicus : CROT-T.

pulsating : *Sulph.*

sitting, while : *Aesc.*, *aloe.*, ammc., am-m., ars., berb., calc.,
cann-s., caust., chel., cocc., cycl., euphr., LYC., *mang.*,
mur-ac., *ph-ac.*, phos., RAT., *ruta.*, sars., SEP., sulph.,
ther., thuj.

amel. : Ans., *ign.*, lach.

sleep, during : Kali-c.

standing agg. : *Aesc.*, arn., ferr., *ign.*

stool, before : Am-c., *berb.*, *carb-an.*, iod., *kali-c.*, lec.,
lach., lil-t., *lyc.*, merc., nat-m., nat-s., nit-ac., nux-v.,
podo., ruta., sulph.

Pain. (CONTD.) :

stool :

during : Aeth., aloe., *alum*., alumn., ambr., am-c., am-m., anac., *ant-c*., asaf., ARS., aur., bac-c., bar-m., bell., *berb*., brom., *bry*., CALC., calc-p., calc-s., canth., caps., carb-an., *carb-s*., *carb-v*., casc., cham., *chel*., chin., chin-a., cimx., COLCH., COLL., coloc., con., crot-t., *cupr*., dros., ferr., ferr-ar., ferr-p., *fl-ac*., GRAPH., grat., hep., hyos., *ign*., *kali-ar*., *kali-bi*., kali-c., kali-p., kali-s., kreos., *lac-c*., *lach*., *lil-t*., LYC., lyss., manc., med., *merc*., merc-i-r., mez., mur-ac., nat-m., NIT-AC., nux-v., *ox-ac*., *paeon*., ph-ac., phos., plant., plat., *plb*., PODO., puls., RAT., rhus-t., sabin., *sanic*., *sep*., SIL., stann., SULPH., sul-ac., sumb., *syph*., tarent., *thuj*., *tub*., *zinc*.

after : AESC., ALOE., alumn., *am-c*., *am-m*., apoc., *ars*., asaf., bar-c., bell., *berb*., bov., *brom*., cact., calc., calc-p., calc-s., canth., carb-s., *carb-v*., carl., casc., caust., cic., cocc., *colch*., crot-t., dios., elaps., *graph*., grat., hydr., IGN., *kali-ar*., kali-bi., kali-c., kali-p. kali-s., *kalm*., *lach*., lil-t., lob., *lyc*., manc., MERC., merc-c., merc-i-r., mez., MUR-AC., *nat-c*., nat-m., nat-p., NIT-AC., *podo*., *psor*., puls., RAT., rhus-t., rhus-v., *ruta*., sabad., *sep*., seneg., sil., staph., stront., SULPH., sul-ac., sumb., tarent., thuj., varat-v.

amel : Acon., *aesc*., aloe., alum., ant-t., arn., asaf., bapt., bry., cahin., calc-p., canth., cham., colch., *coloc*., corn., dulc., *gamb*., hell., lept., nat-s., nuph., NUX-V., RHUS-T., sanic.

straining at, after : *Aesc*., lach., med., nux-v., plb., ruta., *sil*., *thuj*.

Pain (CONTD.) :

urination, during : Rhus-t.

walking, while : CAUST., cycl., *ign.*, mez., ran-s., sep., sulph., sumb.

warm bathing agg. : Brom.

amel. : *Ars., lach., mur-ac., rat.*

extending to abdomen : Aloe., *mez.*, zinc.

genitals : Carb-an., rhod., *sep.*

before stool : Carb-an.

umblicus : *Lach.*

urethra, through : Hipp.

vulva : Ars.

Perineum ; Alum., ant-c., aur., *berb.*, bov., cal-p., *canth.*, carb-an., CAUST., chel., cupr-ar., *cycl.*, kali-bi., *lyc.*, nux-v., phos., plb., *puls.*, selen., sulph., thuj.

urging to urinate : Ant-t., aran., cop.

biting : Agar., alum., ambr., bar-c., canth., caps., carb-v., caust., chin., dulc., hell., kali-c., lach., led., lyc., merl., mez., nat-c , nux-v., ph-ac., phos., rhod., sabin., sep., *sulph.*

burning : Abies-c., AESC., aeth., AGAR., ALOE., *alum.*, ambr., am-c., *am-m.*, ant-c., *apis.*, apoc., arg-n., arn., *ars.*, ars-i., arum-t., aspar., aur., aur-m., bapt., *bar-c.*, bar-m., bell., BERB., bor., *bov., bry.*, cahin., CALC., cal-p., calc-s., canth., CAPS., CARB-AN., CARB-S., CARB-V., card-m., carl., *cast.*, caust., cham., *chel.*, chin., chin-a., clem., cocc., coc-c., *coch.*, coff., colch., coll., *coloc.*, con., *cop., crot-t.*, cub., cupr., cycl.,

Pain, Perineum, burning :

der., dig., dor., *dulc.*, erig., *euph.*, *eup-per.*, ferr., ferr-ar., ferr-i., ferr-p., *gamb.*, gels., GRAPH., grat., ham., hell., *hep.*, hydrc., hyos., ign., *iod.*, ip., IRIS., jug-r., KALI-AR., kali-bi., KALI-C., kali-n., kali-p., KALI-S., *lach.*, lact., laur., *lit-t.*, *lyc.*, lyss., *mag-m.*, mag-s., *manc.*, med., MERC., *merc-c.*, merc-i-f., merc-sul., merl., *mez.*, *mur-ac.*, naja., NAT-A., *nat-c.*, NAT-M., nat-p., nat-s., nicc., NIT-AC., nuph., NUX-V., ol-an., *olnd.*, *op.*, *paeon.*, *petr.*, petros., ph-ac., *phos.*, plat., *plb.*, *prum.*, *psor.*, ptel., PULS., *rat.*, rheum., rhus-t., rhus-v., sabad., salin., sars., SEP., SIL., sin-a., *spong.*, stann., staph., *stront.*, SULPH., *sul-ac.*, sumb., tarent., tep., *ter.*, THUJ., urt-u., verat., varat-v., *zinc.*

daytime, walking while : Nat-m.

morning : Carb-ac., colch., hyper., mag-m., MUR-AC., nicc., NIT-AC., *sulph.*, thuj.

bed, in : Colch.

noon : Dios.

afternoon : coloc., euph., *sulph.*

sleeping, after : Chin.

2 p.m : Dios.

evening : Bar-c., *carb-an.*, iod., kali-c., *mur-ac.*, nit-ac., *sulph.*, thuj., zinc.

night : Am-c., ant-c., *ars.*, iod., nat-m., nit-ac., ox-ac., puls., SULPH.

midnight, before : Thuj.

stool, after : Op.

cold application amel. : *Aloe.*, apis, euph., *kali-c.*, *ter.*

constant : Ars., *kali-c.*, nat-m.

Pain, burning :

diarrhoea, during : ALOE., alum., *ars.*, *aur.*, aur-m., bov., bry., canth., CAPS., carb-an., caust., chin., chin-a., *dulc.*, *gamb.*, glon., graph., grat., IRIS., jug-c., *kali-ar.*, *kali-c.*, kali-s., *lach.*, *manc.*, MERC., *mur-ac.*, *nuph.*, op., *rat.*, SULPH.

after : *Canth.*, *dulc.*, grat., laur., nicc., op., *rat.*

dysentery, in : Aloe., *ars.*, CAPS., *carb-v.*, *coloc.*, *lach.*, **urt-u.**

exercise, after : Sulph.

fissure, in : GRAPH.

flatus, after : *Agar.*, ALOE., ant-t., bapt., *carb-v.*, cham., cocc., dios., phos., plb., psor., *puls.*, *staph.*, *sulph.*, sumb., *teucr.*, *zinc.*

heat agg. : *Iod.*

amel. : *Ars.*

lying, while : *Puls.*

menses, during : Berb., carb-v., zinc.

after : Graph.

moving, after : Crot-t., kali-n.

paroxysmal : Colch., *puls.*

pregnancy, during : *Caps.*

pressure amel : Kali-c.

prolapsed, in the : *Apis.*

rhagades : GRAPH.

rubbing, after : Carb-v., phel., *sabad.*

sitting, while : Ip., SULPH., thuj.

standing, while : *Lach.*, ter.

stool, before : *Berb.*, dios., iod., jug-c., **nat-m.**, **olnd.**, **rat.**, sabad., *sulph.*, verat.

Pain. burning, stool :

during : Agar., *aloe*., ALUM., am-c., am-m., ARS., bar-c., bar-m., *berb*., *bor*., *bry*., *calc*., calc-s., cann-s., *canth*., caps., carb-an., *carb-s*., carb-v., cast., caust., cham., chin., chin-a., chion., clem., cob., cocc., coloc., CON., conn., crot-t., cycl., dios., ferr., ferr-ar., ferr-p., *fl-ac*., gamb., *graph*., grat., hep., *hydr*., IRIS., kali-ar., kali-bi., kali-c., kali-p., kali-s., *lach*., lit-t., *lyc*., mag-m., *merc*., *merc-c*., *merc-sul*., *mur-ac*., nat-a., nat-c., *nat-m*., nat-p., *nat-s*., nicc., OP., osm., phos., phys., pic-ac., *plat*., plb., *puls*., *rat*., rheum., rhus-t., sabad., sep., *sil*., sin-a., *staph*., stram., *stront*., SULPH., *sul-ac*., tab., tep., ter., *verat*., vinc., *zinc*.

after : AESC., agar., ALOE., alumn., am-c., am-m., ant-t., *apis*., ARS., ars-i., arund., asc-t., aster., bar-c., bar-m., *berb*., bov., BRY., *calc*., cann-s., *canth*., caps., *carb-s*., *carb-v*., *carl*., *cast*., CAUST., cic., clem., cob., coc-c., *coloc*., cop., *corn*., crot-t., dirc., dulc., euphr., ferr., ferr-ar., ferr-i., ferr-p., GAMB., *graph*., grat., hell., hep., *hydr*., ign., ind., cod., *iris*., jug-c., jug-r., *kali-ar*., *kali-bi*., *kali-c*., kali-n., kali-p., kali-s., kalm., *lach*., laur., *lit-t*., *lyc*., *mag-c*., *mag-m*., merc., *merc-c*., *mur-ac*., *nat-a*., *nat-c*., *nat-m*., nat-p., *nat-s*., nicc., NIT-AC., nuph., nux-m., *nux-v*., *olnd*., osm., paeon., *petr*., phel., *phos*., pic-ac., ptel., puls., RAT., rheum., rhod., rhus-t., sars., sec., sep., SIL., sin-a., sol-t-ae., stann., *staph*., *stront*., SULPH., tarent., ter., thuj., trom., urt-u., *zinc*.

amel : Clem.

Pain, burning, stool :

        after a hard : Aesc., agar., *aloe.*, alumn., am-m., *ars.*, coc-c., *kali-bi.*, kali-c., lil-t., lyc., mag-m., nat-c., *nat-m.*, phos., RAT., sabad., sec., SIL., *sulph.*, til., ter., thuj.

        tickling : *Ran-s.*

        urination, after : *Nit-ac.*

        vexation agg. : *Cham.*, nat-m.

        walking, while : *Carb-an.*, *mez.*, nat-m., sulph., *thuj.*

        perineum : Ant-c., mur-ac., nit-ac., plb., *rhod.*, sil., thuj.

    coition, after : Sil.

    clawing squeezing, as from a claw in anus : *Ferr.*, lach., nat-c., phel.

        stool, during : Aeth., *thuj.*, zinc.

    cutting : Aesc., aloe, ALUM., *ars.*, calad., calc., calc-p., canth., carb-v., *caust.*, *chel.*, con., *graph.*, *ign.*, indg., *kali-ar.*, *kali-c.*, kali-s., laur., *lyc.*, mag-c., mang., meli., *merc.*, mur-ac., nat-a., nat-c., nat-h., *nit-ac.*, NUX-V., *phos.*, plan., plat., *rat.*, sars., sec., sep., SIL., stann., staph., *sulph.*, sumb., thuj., zinc.

        morning : Graph., mang.

            bed, in : *Graph.*

            rising, after : Mang.

        forenoon, walking, while : *Sulph.*

        afternoon : Sep., sulph.

        evening : Nat-h., phos.

        night : Sep.

            10 a. m. : Aloe.

Pain, cutting :
  diarrhoea, during : ARS.
  dysentery in : *Merc-c.*
  sitting : RAT.
  standing agg. : *Lach.*
  stool, before : *Asar.*, sep., sulph., verat-v.
    during : Agar., all-c., alum., am-c., ant-t., ars., canth., carb-v., dios., *mur-ac.*, nat-a., nat-c., *nat-m.*, nat-p., NIT-AC., *phos.*, *pic-ac.*, *plat.*, plb., *puls.*, sars., sep., stann., SULPH., sumb., vib.
    after : *Aesc.*, agar., *aloe.*, calc., chel., NIT-AC., NUX-V., pic-ac., *puls.*, RAT., sin-a., staph., sumb.
  walking, while : Mag-c., meli., *sulph.*
  extending up rectum : Hell., *sep.*, *sulph.*
  Perineum : Am-m., aur., bov., lyc., nux-v., thuj.
    morning : Lyc.
    evening : Am-m.
  drawing : Ant-c., aur-s., calc., cann-s., carb-v., chel., chil., *cycl.*, eupc. kreos., lach., lact., mang., mez., phos., rhod., zinc.
    coition, after : Caust.
    downwards : Phos.
    sitting, while : Chin., *cycl.*
    walking, while : *Cycl.*
    extending into abdomen : Aloe, zinc.
      through genitals : Carb-an., rhod.
        before stool : Carb-an.
      to umbilicus : *Lach.*
      upwards : Mez., plb., thuj.
      urethra, through : Hipp.

Pain :

    grawing : Carb-v., elaps., ferr., merc., phos., stann.

    griping: *Calc*., carb-v., *cocc*., IGN., kali-i., mur-ac., nat-m.,
        nit-ac., ox-ac., thuj.

        forenoon : *Calc*.

        afternoon : *Cocc*.

        evening : Mez.

        driving, while : Glon.

        sitting : *Calc*., *cocc*.

        stool, when not at : barb-v.

        amel : *Nat-a*.

        extending to abdomen : Mez.

    lancinating (See Cutting).

    pinching : Eug., merc., nat-m., *nat-ac*.
        in Perineum : *Puls*.

    pressing (pressure): Acon., AESC., *aloe*., alum., ang., ant-c.,
        apoc., arg-m., *arn*., *ars*., asf., *bar-c*., bar-m., *bell*.,
        berb., bry., cact., cahin., calc., *calc-s*., carb., carb-s.,
        carb-v., CAUST., chel., *chin*., chin-a., cob., coll.,
        coloc., con., cop., *crot-t*., *cycl*., dulc., eug., eup-pur.,
        ferr-i., form., gran., *graph*., hell., hydr., IGN., iod., *iris*.,
        kali-ar., *kali-bi*., kali-c., *kali-n*., kali-p., kali-s., kreos.,
        lach., lact., laur., LIT-T., *lyc*., mag-c., *mag-m*., *merc*.,
        merc-i-f., merl., mez., *murx*., mur-ac., nat-c., nat-m.,
        NIT-AC., NUX-V., op., ox-ac., PETR., phel., *phos*.,
        plat., ptel., *puls*., rhus-t., *sars*., seneg., *sep*., sil., spig.,
        stann., staph., stry., SULPH., valer., verat., verb.,
        zinc.

        morning : *Kali-bi*.

        forenoon : Kali-bi.

Pain, pressing :

    noon : Agar., kali-bi.

    afternoon : chel., cycl., sluph.

        sleep, during : Cycl.

    evening : Chin-s., ran-s.

        bed, in : Iod.

    night : *Lyc.*,

    diarrhoea would come on, as if : *Crot-t.*, mag-c.

        as in a : Calc., nat-m.

    downward, outward, etc. : Agar., *aloe.*, berb., bry., calc-p., cann-s., *carb-v.*, cimic., cob., *conn.*, CROT-T., dios., dros., *ip.*, kali-n., *lach.*, lil-t., lyc., mag-c., *nit-ac.*, *nux-m.*, nux-v., ox-ac., pic-ac., PODO., *puls.*, SULPH., verat.

    faeces were lodged in rectum, as if : *Caust.*

    flatus, during : *Carb-v.*

    lying, while : Crot-t.

    menses, before : Ign., petr.

        during : *Aloe.*

    mental exertion : Caust.

    motion agg. : *Nux-v.*

    sitting, while : Amm-c., calc., *cann-s.*, *cycl.*, euphr., sulph., thuj.

    standing, while : Arn., *ferr.*

    stool, before : Ant-c., cob., *nat-m.*, *nit-ac.*, *nux-v.*, PLAT. sul-ac., til.

        during : Alum., asaf., conn., *kali-bi.*, lil-t., LYC., nat-m., ox-ac., *podo.*, sin-a., SULPH., *zinc.*

        after : Apoc., *calc.*, caust., *ign.*, *kali-bi.*, *kalm.*, *merc.*, nit-ac., ph-ac., phos., plat., *podo.*, *puls.*, seneg., sil., sul-ac., *sulph.*

Pain, pressing, stool :

      not for : *Dros.*, *LACH.*, mez.

   walking : *Cycl* , *ran-s.*, sulph.

perineum : *Alum.*, *asaf.*, *lyc.*, sulph., thuj.

rasping : Ant-c., grat., nat-m., verat.

scraping : Ant-c., calc-p., crot-t., grat., nat-m., puls., verat.

stooling (See Stitching).

smarting (See Burning).

soreness : AESC., *agar.*, agn., ALOE., alum., ambr., am-c.,
     am-m., ant-c., ant-s., APIS., arn., *ars.*, aspar. , aur.,
     bar-c., BAR-M., BELL., BERB., *bry.*, *calc.*, *calc-p.*,
     calc-s., *caps* , *carb-an.*, *carb-s.*, *carb-v.*, CAUST.,
     coloc., crot-t., *cycl.*, dios., elaps., gal-ac., GAMB.,
     GRAPH., HAM., hep., IGN., IRIS., KALI-AR.,
     kali-bi., KALI-C., *kali-p.*, KALI-S., LACH., lact.,
     lil-t., LYC., MERC., *merc-c.*, merc-i-f., merc-sul.,
     MUR-AC., nat-a., nat-c., *nat-m.*, nat-s., nat-p., NIT-
     AC., nux-m., *nux-v.*, PAEON., petr., ph-ac., phos.,
     phys., *podo.*, prun., psor., PULS., RAT., *rhus-t.*, sars.,
     sep., SIL., sol-t-ae., spong., stam., staph., SULPH.,
     sul-ac., syph., tab., thuj., verat., vib., *zinc.*, zing.

     morning : Calc-p., thuj.

     evening : Bar-c., *carb-an.*, kali bi., *sulph.*, zinc.

     night : Phel., sars.

     lying on back : Chel.

     menses during : Berb., carb-v.

     moving, after : Crot-t., *puls*.

     sitting, while : *Am-m.*, *berb.*, CAUST., chel., *cycl.*,
       mag-c., *mur-ac.*, RAT., *sulph.*

Pain, soreness.

    stool, during : Aesc., agar., ALOE., ALUM., *ant-c.*, brach., caust., coloc., *graph.*, *grat.*, nat-c., *nat-m* , *sulph.*

    hard, during : *Nat-m.*, *sulph.*

    after : *Aesc.*, ALOE., *alum.*, ant-c., APIS., apoc., cal-s., *carb-s.*, *cham.*, chel., colch., crot., gamb., GRAPH., hep., IGN., iod., kali-bi., kali-c., mag-m., *merc.*, mez., *mur-ac.*, *nat-m.*, NIT-AC., nux-m., nux-v., phos., podo., puls., RAT., stann., staph., *sulph.*

    diarrhoeic, after : Nat-m., phel., SULPH., tab.

    walking, while : Arg-m., CAUST., cycl., *kali-bi.*, *mez.*, *nit-ac.*

    perineum : Alum., echi.

  splinter, like a : *Aesc.*, agar., *alum.*, *arg-n.*, bar-c., *carb-v.*, coll., NIT-AC., RAT., *sil.*, sulph.

  sticking : AESC , aloe., ant-c., *ars.*, cact., calc., *carb-v.*, CAUST., chel., *coll.*, *coloc.*, ferr-c., GRAPH., grat., IRIS., jac-c., kali-c., kali-n., lact., lyc., nat-m., *nit-ac.*, NUX-V., phos., puls., *rat.*, rumx., *sil.*, SULPH., sumb., *teucr.*, *thuj.*

    stool, during : Ferr-i., NIT-AC.

    after : NUX-V., RAT.

  perineum : Alum., bell., bov., carb-v., mag-m., merc., sep., thuj.

  stinging : AESC., acon., *am-m.*, *apis.*, *ars.*, *caps.*, carb-an., *caust.*, coch., lyc., mag-m., *nat-m.*, NUX-V., *phos.*, puls., sil., *staph.*, sulph.

    night, lying : ARS., puls.

Pain, stinging :

    menses, during : Phos.

    stool, during : Berb., caps., caust., coc-c., ip., *lyc.*, mag-m., nat-c., nat-m., nicc., NIT-AC., *sil.*, sulph.

        after : Aloe., berb., *canth.*, kali-n., NIT-AC., *puls.*, *sulph.*

    walking, while : Carb-an.

    stitching : *Acon.*, AESC., agar., *all-c.*, aloe., alum., alumn., am-m., ang., ant-t., *apis.*, arg-n., arn., ARS., arund., aur., aur-s., *bar-c.*, *bar-m.*, bell., *benz-ac.*, *berb.*, bor., bov., brom., bry.. cact., calad., *culc..* calc-p., calc-s., cann-i., cann-s., canth., *caps.*, CARB-AN., *carb-s.*, *carb-v.*, carl., CAUST., cham., chel., chin., chin-a., coc-c., colch., coloc., CON., *cop.*, *croc.*, crot-t., cycl., euphr., ferr-ar., ferr-i., ferr-ma., gins., *graph.*, grat., IGN., indg., ip., jac-c., jatr., kali-ar., kali-bi., KALI-C., kali-n., kali-p., KALI·S., kreos., LACH., led., LYC., lyss., mag-c., *mag-m.*, *mag-p.*, *med.*, meli., MERC., merc-c., merc-i-f., *mez.*, mosch., *mur-ac.*, *nat-c.*, *nat-m.*, nicc., NIT-AC., nuph., nux-m., nux-v., ol-an., petr., phel., *ph-ac.*, *phos.*, *phyt.*, plat., plb., *plus.*, ran-b., ran-s., *rat.*, *rhus-t.*, *ruta.*, *sabad.*, SEP., SIL., spong., stann., stram., stry., SULPH., *sul-ac.*, tarent., teucr., *thuj.*, *til.*, zinc.

    morning : Lyc., mag-c.,

        waking, after : mag-c. zinc,

    forenoon : Lach.

    afternoon : Agar., chin-s., lyc., nat-m., sulph.

    evening : Benz-ac., bor., cal-p., carb-s., carb-v., gran., iris., merc-c., nat-m., nit-ac., SULPH., thuj., zinc.

Pain, sitching :

      bed, in : *Nat-m*.

night : Sep., thuj., stry.

      midnight : Thuj.

alternating with burning in prepuce : Thuj.

      with itching in glans penis : Thuj.

coition, during : Calc.

coughing, on : *Ign.*, LACH , nit-ac.

dinner, after : Phos.

eating, before : *Caust*.

      after : NUX-V.

erect, when body is : PETR.

flatus, on passing : Bry., phos.

      amel : Coloc., *mag-c*.

itching : Alum., bry., coloc., stann., sulph.

lying, while : Nat-c., SULPH.

menses, during : Aloe., *ars*., phos.

mental exertion, after : NUX-V.

perio dicol : Agar., *ign*.

pregnancy, during : *Kali-c*.

sitting while : *Ars*., *calc*., gran., kali-c., nat-c., *ru'a*., SULPH., *thuj*.

sneezing, when : *Lach*.

standing, while : *Sulph*., valer.

stool, before : Asar., *berb*., *con*., gamb., *kali-c*., phos., plat., spong., sul-ac.

      during : Am-c., am-m., *berb*., calc-s., carb-an., carb-s., *carb-v*., caust., chin., coc-c., ferr-i., GRAPH., *ign*., ip.,

Pain, stitching, stool during.

    laur., mag-m., *nat-c.*, nat-m., NIT-AC., nux-m., *nux-v.*, pic-ac., *sep.*, *staph.*, sul-ac.

    hard, during : Bar-c., bell., prun., sulph.

    after : *Aloe.*, am-m., *berb.*, calad., canth., cham., kali-n., laur., *lyc.*, mag-m., *mez.*, nat-m., nicc., NIT-AC., pic-ac., *plat.*, *rat.*, sep., stann., thuj.

        difficult, stool, after : Alum., *plat.*, *rat.*

  urination, during : Carb-s., sulph.

  walking, while : *Ars.*, coc-c., crot-t., meli., nat-p., petr., *sil.*, squil., sulph., zinc.

    after : Thuj.

  in open air amel : Thuj.

extending to abdomen : Aloe , mag-m., *sep.*

    back : Carb.

    bladder : Mosch., thuj.

    downwards and outwards : *Carb-v.*, lith.

    genitals, to, while walking : Sil.

    ilium and glans penis : Petr., *thuj.*

    inguinal region, left : Croc., kreos.

    inner side of thigh : Alum.

    loins : Aloe.

    outward : *Carb-v.*, lith.

    penis : Carl.

    pudendum, during menses : Aloe.

        after stool : Cast.

    root of penis : Zinc.

    upward : Aesc., *graph.*, IGN., *lach.*, mag-c., *mez.*, *rhus-t.*, *sep.*, thuj.

    stool, after : Alum., *mez.*, sulph.

Pain, stitching, extending to :
    urethra : Carb-s., cocc., thuj.
    Perineum : Alum., Am-m., aur., berb., bov., *calc-p.*,
        carb-v., chel., chin., mag-m., merc., nit-ac., sep , spig.,
        sulph., thuj.
        evening : Am-m., sep.
        extending to **anus** : Nit-ac.
            penis : *Calc-p*.
            uterus : Berb.
tearing : *All-c.*, alumn., aur., *berb.*, calc , carb-s., carb-v.,
        chin., *colch.*, erig., eupi., ferr., grat., ign., *kali-c.*,
        kreos., lach., laur., led., *lyc.*, *mez.*, nat-m., NIT-AC.,
        NUX-V., ph-ac., phos., *ruta.*, sars., sep., sulph., sul-ac.,
        thuj., zinc.
    morning : Ph-ac.
    evening : Ph-ac.
    after hard stool : Lyc.
    bed, in : Chin.
    bending forward amel : Alumn.
    coughing, on : Lach.
    dinner, after : Mang.
    lying on back amel : Alumn.
    moving, on : Valer.
    sitting, while : *Ruta*.
    stool, during : Agar., *calc.*, colch., ferr., *lach.*, nat-a.,
        NAT-M., *nit-ac.*, sars., *sel.*, *sep.*, *sul-ac.*
        after : Aesc., alumn., *kali-c.*, lyc., nat-m., NIT-AC.
    twitching : Thuj.
    urinating, while : *Ruta*.
    extending into abdomen : Mag-c.

Pain, tearing, extending :

    during stool : Mag-c.

    upward : *Lach.*, sep.

    Perineum : Am-m., mez.

    tenesmus : Acon., AESC., agar., ALOE., alum., ambr., am-c., *anac.*, ant-c., APIS., apoc., *arg-m.*, *arn.*, *ars.*, ars-i., arum-t., asaf., atro., aur-m., bar-c., bar-m., *bell.*, benz., berb., *bov.*, brom., bry., cact., *calc.*, calc-s., *canth.*, CAPS., carb-an., carb-s., *carb-v.*, *caust.*, cham., chin-s., cob., cocc., COLCH., *coll.*, *coloc.*, con., *corn.*, *crot-t.*, cupr., cupr-ar., *cycl.*, der., dig., dios., circ., *euph.*, eup-per., eupi., fago., ferr., ferr-ar., ferr-i., ferr-m., ferr-p., gamb., gels., graph., grat., *ham.*, hep., hyos., ign., iod., *ip.*, iris., kali-ar., *kali-bi.*, kali-c., *kali-i.*, *kali-n.*, kreos., *lach.*, lac-c., lact., laur., LIL-T., *lyc.*, lycps., *lyss.*, mag-s., manc., MERC., MERC-C., merc-cy., *mez.*, mill., mur-ac., *nat-a.*, *nat-c.*, *nat-m.*, nat-p., nicc., NIT-AC., nux-m., *nux-v.*, oena., ol-an., op., ox-ac., petr., phel., ph. ac., phos., phys., *phyt.*, pic-ac., *plat.*, plb., podo., psor., ptel., puls., rat., rheum., rhod., rhus-t., rumx., ruta., sang., sel., senec., *sep.*, *sil.*, sol-n., sol-t-ae., spig., spong., squil., stann., STAPH., *stront.*, SULPH., sumb., tab., tarent., ter., thuj., trom., verat., verat-v., vip., zinc.

    morning : Aeth ; nicc.

        rising, after : Aeth.

    evening : Ferr., plat.

    night : Bov., *merc.* zinc.

    bladder, and : Alum., CAPS., lil-t., *merc-c.*, NUX-V.

    coffee, after : *Nat-m.*

    constipation, during : Asaf., *con.*, plb., *nux-v.*, vib.

    diarrhoea, before : Hydr.

Pain, tenesmus, diarrhoea :

        during : *Alum.*, ARS., carb-s., carb-v., cimic., *colec.*, cop., corn., crot-t., form., *gamb.*, hydr., mag-m., mag-s., *merc.*, MERC-C., *nit-ac.*, op., phys., phyt., plb., ptel., sarr., sel., *sulph.*, tab.

        after : *Dulc.*, hydr., laur., *lil-t.*, mag-c., phel., phos., rhus-t., stront., tab.

    dinner, after : Alum., nat-m.

    dysentery, during : Acon., APIS., arn., ars-i., CAPS., COLCH., con., cop., dios., ip., *merc.*, MERC-C., *nit-ac.*, rheum., sulph., ter., xan.

    eating : *Colcc.*, crot-t.

    flatus, on attempting to suppress : Acon.

    hard stool, with : *Con.*

    menses, before : Thuj.

        during : *Am-c.*, nat-s.

    milk, after : Nicc.

    sitting, while : Crot-t., *sulph.*

    stool, before : Acon., aeth., AGAR., alum., arn., berb., cham., coloc., crot-c., dirc., fago., grat., mag-m., *merc.*, MERC-C., *nux-v.*, phys., plat., plb., sep., SULPH., tarent., verat.

        during : ACON., aesc., *aeth.*, ALOE., AGAR., alum., am-c., am-m., ang., ant-t., apis., apoc., arg-n., *arn.*, *ars.*, arum-t., asc-t., aster., bapt., *bell.*, calc., calc-s., canth., *caps.*, carb-ac., carb-s., *caust.*, cedr., cob., coff-t., *colch.*, *coll.*, *coloc.*, con.. cop., *corn.*, crot-t., *cupr.*, dios., fago., ferr., ferr-ar., ferr-m., fl-ac., form., gamb., gran., graph., grat., hell., hep., hipp., hydr., hyper., IP., iris., kali-ar., kali-bi., kali-chl., kali-i., kali-n., kalm., lach., *lac-c.*, laur., *lil-t.*, lob-s., lyc., lyss., *mag-c.*, mag-m., mang., MERC., MERC-C., *morph.*, myric., *nat-a.*, *nat-c.*, *nat-m.*, *nat-s.*, nicc.,

Pain, tenesmus, stool, during :

> *nit-ac.*, NUX-V., OP., ox-ac., petr., phys., phyt., pic-ac., plan., plat., plb., *podo.*, ptel., rob., rhus-t., senec., sep., *spong.*, staph., *sulph.*, tab., ther., thuj., *trom.*, verat., zinc.

> after: *Aeth.*, AGAR., ambr., am-m., ant-t., *apis.*, apoc., ars., aster., bapt., *bell.*, bov., calc-p., cals-s., *canth.*, *caps.*, cob., *cocc.*, *colch.*, corn., cupr-ac., dios., dros., dulc., erig., fago., fl-ac., gamb., gins., grat., hell., *ign.*, ind., indg., ip., jug-c., kali-ar., *kali-bi.*, kali-c., kali-n., kali-p., *kali-s.*, lach., laur., lil-t., lyc., lyss., *mag-c.*, *mag-m.*, mag-s., manc., MERC., MERC-C., merc-i-r., *mez.*, *nat-m.*, nicc., phel., PULS., *rheum.*, *rhus-t.*, sars., SULPH., tab., *trom.*, zinc.

> amel : Acon., aesc., aloe., alum., ant-t., arn., ars., asaf., bapt., bov., bry., cahin., cal-p., canth.. cham., colch., *coloc.*, corn., dulc., GAMB., hell., lept., nat-s., nuph., NUX-V., RHUS-T., sanic., tarent.

urination, during : Carb-v., ferr., med., *prun.*

> after : Coloc., mur-ac.

walking, while : *Sulph.*

warmth amel : Coloc., sulph.

water, on hearing running : LYSS.

extending to bladder : Canth., *caps.*, *med.*, merc-c., *nux-v.*

> perineum : Mez.

> urethra : Mez.

twinging : Caust., kali-c., lact., lyc., mag-c., nat-c., zinc.

exercise, after : Coc-c.

flatus amel : Kali-bi.

stool, during : Spong.

> after : Canth., grat.

writhing in anus : *Cnoc.*

Paralysis (See Inactivity) : Acon., aeth., agar., aloe., *alum.*, arn., ars., ars-i., atro., *bar-m.*, *bell.*, bry., *calc.*, caust., chin., chin-a, coll., coloc., cupr., ferr., *gels.*, *graph.*, *hyos.*, kali-ar., kali-c., kali-p., laur., manc., MUR-AC., nat-m., ph-ac., PHOS., PLB., puls., rhus-t., SEC., scl., SIL., sulph., tab., tarent., thuj., verat.

sensation of : ALOE., graph., kali-c., petr., ph-ac., sabad.

Perspiration about the anus and perineum : Agar., *alum.*, bell., carb-an., con., *hep.*, kali-c., psor., rhus-t., thuj.

morning : *Thuj.*

night : Kali-c.

Plug were pressing out, sensation as if : Bry., *crot-t.*, kali-bi., *lach.*, lil-t., *sep.*, *sil.*

sensation of, wedged between pubis and coccyx : Aloe.

Polypi : Am-m., *calc.*, *cal-p.*, kali-br., *nit-ac.*, nux-v., PHOS., ruta., sang., teucr.

Prickling : Agar., bry., cact., colch., grat., lact., NIT-AC., *ter.*

stool, during : Cact.

after : Grant.

Prolapsus : *Aesc.*, all-c., alumn., ant-c., APIS., apoc., arn., *ars.*, *asar.*, aur., *bell.*, bufo., CALC., *calc-s.*, canth., *carb-s.*, caust., cic., cocc., *colch.*, *coll.*, *crot-c.*, crot-t., *dig.*, dios., *dulc.*, elaps., *ferr.*, ferr-ar., *ferr-i.*, ferr-p., fl-ac., *gamb.*, *gels.*, gran., *graph.*, *hep.*, *hydr.*, IGN., iris., *kali-bi.*, kali-n., *lach.*, *lyc.*, *mag-m.*, *mang.*, med., MERC., *merc-c.*, mez., MUR-AC., *nat-m*, *nat-s.*, *nit-ac.*, nux-m., NUX-V., *phos.*, phyt., *plb.*, PODO.,

Prolapsus:

    psor., rhus-t., *ruta.*, SEP., *sil.*, sol-t-ae., *sulph.*, sumb., syph., tab., ther., thuj., valer.. zinc.

morning : Podo.

forenoon : Rhus-t.

evening : IGN.

night : *Aesc.*

children : *Ferr., hydr., nux-v.*, PODO.

convulsive : *Ars*.

diarrhoea, during : *Calc.*, DULC., gamb., mag-m., MERC., *mur-ac.*, PODO.

flatus, when passing : Valer.

haemorrhage of rectum, after : *Ars.*

kneeling : Ail.

menses, during : Aur., podo.

mental excitement, from : Podo.

painful : *Ars.*, ther.

parturition, after : *Podo., ruta.*

sitting agg. : Ther.

smoking agg. : *Sep*.

sneezing, after : Podo.

standing : *Ferr-i.*

stool, before : *Podo., ruta.*

during : *Ant-c.*, ail., asar., bell., bry., *cinnb., calc.*, colch., crot-t., dulc., ferr., ferr-ar., ferr-p., *fl-ac., gamb.*, IGN., kali-n., LYC., mag-m., mez., mur-ac., *nux-v.*, plan., PODO., *rhus-t., ruta.*, SEP., *sulph.*, trom.

after : *Aesc.*, ant-c., apoc., ars., asar.. canth., carb-v., *cocc.* crot-t., euph., *hep., ign., indg.*, iris., kali-bi., *lach., merc.*, mez., mur-ac., **nat-m., nit-ac.**, *phos.*, plat., PODO., *sep.*, sol-t-ae., *sulph., trom.*

Prolapsus :
    stooping, on : Ruta.
    straining, without : *Graph.*, *ruta.*
    urination, during : MUR-AC., *valer.*
    difficult : *Sep.*
    vomiting, when : *Mur-ac.*, *podo.*
    sensation of : *Aesc.*, chel., dios., iris.
Pulsation : Aloe., alum., alumn., am-m., apis., benz., berb.,
        cal-p., caps., caust., crot-t., cycl., grat., *ham.*, LACH.,
        lyss., manc., meli., *nat-m.*, rhod., seneg., *sulph.*
    evening : Am-m.
        sitting, amel in bed : Am-m.
    menses, during : Lach., *lyss.*
    sitting, while : *Aloe.*, am-m.
    small hammers, like : LACH.
    stool, during : Nat-m.
        after : Aloe, alumn,, apis., berb., caps., *lach.*, manc.,
        sang., seneg., *sulph.*
    Perineum : Bov., *caust.*, polyg.
Recedes, stool : (See Constipation).
Redness of anus : Aloe, ars, cham., nat-m., *petr.*, SULPH.,
        valer., *zing.*
Relaxed anus : ALOE, APIS., apoc., *carb-v.*, chin., kali-c.,
        kali-p., *petr.*, PHOS., puls., rhod., *sec.*, zing.
    sensation of, after stool : Lept., podo.
Retraction : Agar., bapt., bry., kali-bi., *op.*, plb., tell.
    painful : *Kali-bi.*
    stool, after : *Kali-bi.*
Sensitive : *Aloe*, *bell.*, berb., calc., *caust.*, *graph.*, *hep.*, *lach.*,
        lil-t., *lyc.*, MAG-M., MUR-AC., NIT-AC., nux-v.,
        podo., rat., *sep.*, sil., sul-ac., syph., thuj.

Shock, electric-like : Apis., stry.

    stool, before : Apis.

Slip back, stools. (See Constipation.)

Slow action of rectum. (See Inactivity.)

Spasms in : *Caust.*, *colch.*, *ferr*., tab.

    coition, during : Merc-c.

    walking : Caust.

    with urging to urinate : *Caust*.

Straining. (See Tenesmus.)

Stricture : *Aesc.*, agar., *aloe.*, alum., ang., *bar-m.*, bell., *bor.*, calc., *calc-sil.*, *camph.*, colch., con., crot-t., elaps., fl-ac., hep., ign., kreos., *lach.*, *lyc.*, med., mez., *nat-m.*, nit-ac., phos., plb., *ruta.*, sec., thuj.

Swelling of anus : *Aesc.*, *apis.*, aur., bell., bor., bufo., *coll.*, crot-t., cur., *graph.*, *hep.*, ign., kali-i., lach., med., mur-ac., nux-v., *paeon.*, *podo.*, phys., sarr., *sulph.*, teucr.

    black : *Carb-v.*, *mur-ac*.

    menses, during : **Sep**.

    sensation of : *Aesc.*, cact., graph., hep., nat-m., nux-m., sulph.

    Raphe of perineum : Thuj.

Tenesmus. (See Pain).

Tension : *Calc.*, chin., euphr., graph., *ign.*, *lyc.*, *nux-v.*, rhus-t., *sep.*, SIL.

    convulsive : Ign.

    stool, after : Berb., sep.

    Perineum : Echi.

Tickling. (See Itching.)

Tingling : *Carb-v.*, *colch.*, ferr-ma., plat., ter.

    evening : Plat.

    stool, during : *carb-v*.

Trembling in anus : con.

Tubercle on Perineum : *Thuj.*

Twitching : Agn., ars., bry., calc., carb-ac., colch., *coloc.*, iod., merc., nat-m., *sil., staph.*

afternoon : Coloc.

bed, in : Chin.

Ulceration : *Alumn., calc.,* caust., CHAM., cub., *hep., hydr.,* kali-c., *kali-i., nat-s., paeon., petr.,* phos., *phyt.,* puls., sars., SIL., staph., syph.

Unnoticed stool : Acon., *aloe.,* ars., carl., colch., coloc., cur., ferr-ma., grat., *hyos., mur-ac.,* ph-ac., *plb., staph.,* tab., verat.

hard stool : ALOE, *coloc.*

thin watery, passes while urinating : *Mur-ac.*

Urging, desire (See Tenesmus). Abort., acon., AESC., aeth., AGAR., all-c., *aloe., alum.,* alumn., *anac., apis,.* arg-m., *arg-n., arn., ars.,* ars-h., ars-i., arum-t., asc-t., asar., atro., aur., aur-m., bar-c., *bell.,* benz-ac., *berb., bism.,* bov., *bry.,* bufo., cadm., cahin., calad., calc., calc-p., camph., cann-s., canth., caps., carb-an., carb-s., carb-v., cast-eq., cast-v., cast., caust., cham., *chel.,* chin., chin-s., cic., *cimx.,* cimic., cist., clem., cob., cocc., coc-c., coff., *colch., coloc.,* com., *con., corn.,* croc., crot-c., crot-t., cupr., cycl., dig., dios., *dulc.,* elaps., eug., fago., ferr., ferr-ar., ferr-i., ferr-ma.. gamb., gent., glon., *graph.,* gran., grat., ham., *hep.,* hydr., hyos., hyper., IGN., indg., iod., iris., kali-bi., *kali-c.,* kali-chl., kali-n., kalm., kreos., lach., lact., LIL-T., lyc., mag-c., mag-m., mag-s., manc., MERC., *merc-c.,* merc-i-f., merc-i-r., mez., naja., nat-a., nat-c., nat-m., nat-p., nat-s., nux-m., NUX-V., oena., *op.,* osm., ox-ac., pall., petr., phel., *phos.,* phys., PIP-M., plan., *plat.,* PLB., *podo.,* prun., ptel., *puls., ran-s.,*

Urging (CONTD.) :

> rat., *rheum.*, *rhod.*, rhus-t., *ruta.*, sabad., sabin., sars., sec., senec., *sep.*, serp., SIL., sol-t-ae., spong., stann., *staph.*, stront., SULPH., sul-ac., sumb., *tab.*, tarent., tell., ther., *thuj.*, trom., verat., verb., vib., vinc., ust., zinc.

> evening in sleep : Phyt.

> night : *Aloe.*, carl., coloc., graph., lyc., mex-i-r., nat-m., phys., SULPH., thuj., zinc.

> menses, before : Mang.

> waking, on : *Aloe.*, ferr-i.

> 11 p.m. : Gels., mag-c., merc-i-r., pip-m.

> midnight : Dios., lach.

absent in company (See Inactivity) : AMBR.

anxious : Acon., *merc.*, *nux-v.*, ol-an.

breakfast, during : Dios.

> after : Carb-s., grat.

clothing, on tightening : Bry.

coffee, after : Nat-m.

coition, after : Nat-p.

colic, during : Coloc., ind., NUX-V.

constant : Aesc., ant-s., arn., ars., asaf., bar-c., berb., bry., calc., cob., con., cop., CROT-T., ham., hyos., *ign.*, kali-a., lil-t., mag-c., mag-m., MERC., MERC-C., *merc-d.*, nat-a., nat-m., *nat-s.*, *nux-v.*, phyt., *pip-m.*, ptel., ruta., sin-n., *sulph.*, sumb., zinc-s.

dinner, during : Dios.

> after : Ant-c., cann-s., caust., colch., coloc., ferr-ma., kali-bi., mag-m., nat-m., par., phel., ran-s., sulph.

Urging (CONTD.) :

    eating, after (See Diarrhoea) : ALOE., anac., apoc., bar-c., cham., clem., COLOC., ferr-ma., fl-ac., phos., *rheum.*, rhus-t., sulph., zinc.

    effort, great desire passes away with : ANAC.

    eructation, on each : Aesc.

    exciting news, after : Gels.

    flatus, when passing : ALOE., spig., ruta.

        passing amel : Caps., *colch.*, mag-c., mez., nat-a., ruta.,

    frequent : Abrot., *ambr.*, *apis.*, *arg-m.*, arn., asaf., BAR-C., bell., berb., bor., brom., cahin., cal-p., carb-an., *caust.*, *coloc.*, CON., CORN., dios., ham., *hep.*, hura., *hyos.*, *ign.*, kreos., lac-c., lac-d., LIL-T., MERC., MERC-C., *nat-m.*, nat-s., nit-ac., NUX-V., ox-ac., petr., ph-a., phos., PLAT., *puls.*, *rheum.*, ruta., sars., stann., stram., sulph., tab.

    fright, from : *Caust.*

    hang down, letting feet : Rhus-t.

    labour pain, with every : Nux-v., plat.

    lying, while : (See Diarrhoea).

    menses, before : Eupi.

        during : Calc., mang.

    motion, on : *Aloe.*

    sitting, on : Crot-t.

    smoking, while : Calad., thuj.

    standing, while : Aloe., bry., lil-t.

    startled, when : *Gels.*

    stool, before : All-s., *aloe.*, berb., calc-f., euphr., ferr-i., fl-ac., grat., hell., kali-n., lact., mez., osm., *podo.*, *rheum.*, *rhus-t.*, stront., SULPH.

Urging, stool :

    during : Abrot., *aesc*., aeth., am-m., anac., ant-c., arg-m., ars-i., bov., bry., calad., calc., carb-s., carl., coca., *coll*., con., cycl., dios., dirc., dros., dulc., eupi., ferr., form., gamb., graph., grat., hep., inul., iris., lycps., merl., mez., nat-c., nat-p., nicc., nit-ac., ox-ac., phys., phyt., pic-ac., pip-m., plam., plat., ptel., ran-s., rat., rhus-t., sars., sep., sil., stann., stram., SULPH., sul-ac., tab., tarent., verb.

    after: Aesc., *aeth*., ALOE., ars., ars-i., bar-c., berb., bry., cal-p., camph., cic., cocc., colch., crot-t., cycl., dig., dios., dros., ferr., ferr-ar., ferr-i., form., grat., ign., iod., iris., kali-p., *lach*., lyc., mag-m., MERC., MERC-C., merc-i-r., naja., nat-a., nat-c., *nat-p*., nicc., *nit-ac*., nux-v., petr., RHEUM., ruta., samb., sol-t-ae., spig., stann., SULPH., tab., til.

not for stool, but : LACH.

rising from : Rheum., rumx.

    after, amel : Acon., aesc., aloe., alum., ant-t., arn., ars., asaf., bapt., bry., cahin., calc-p., canth., cham., colch., *coloc*., corn., dulc., GAMB., gels., hell., lept., nat-s., nuph., NUX-V., RHUS-T., sanic., tarent.

    sudden : Aesc., agar., *aloe*., ant-s., bar-c., bry., carb-v., cic., cocc., CROT-T., cycl., dig., dirc., *ferr*., gent., graph., ign., kali-bi., kali-n., lac-ac., *lach*., lil-t., mag-m., manc., naja., *nat-c*., *nat-p*., *nat-s*., plat., *podo*., *psor*., ptel., rhus-t., rob., sep., SULPH., sumb., tab., verat., zinc.

        after : *Cann-s*.

        morning : Manc., SULPH.

        evening : Gent.

Urging, stool :

     night : Nux-v.

supper, after : Calc-p., ox-ac., podo.

thinking about it, on : Iris., *ox-ac.*

tormenting, but not for stool : *Lach.*

urination, during : ALOE., alum., aphis., cann-s., *canth.,*
    caust., crot-h., cycl., dig., merc., *mur-ac.,* NUX-V.,
    prun., *puls.,* squil., staph., sumb., thuj.

    amel : Nat-m.

    after : Cann-s.

urine is discharged, but only : Lil-t.

vertigo, during : Spig.

walking, while : Cob., coloc., laur., pall., rheum.

water, on hearing running : LYSS.

Warts (See Condylomata).

HOMŒOPATHIC BOOKS FOR ALL

ALLEN, H.C.
Key Notes with Nosodes — Rs. 7.00
The Materia Medica of the Nosodes — Rs. 25.00

ALLEN, T.F.
Boenninghausen's Therapeutic
Pocket Book — Rs. 13.00

BERNOVILLE, FORTIER
What We Must Not Do in
Homoeopathy — Rs. 3.50

BIDWELL, G.I.
How To Use The Repertory — Rs. 5.50

BOGER, C.M.
Synoptic Key to Materia Medica — Rs. 11.00
Additions to Kent's Repertory — Rs. 2.50

BOERICKE & DEWEY
The Twelve Tissue Remedies of
Schussler — Rs. 9.50

BOERICKE, W.
Pocket Manual of Homoeopathic
Materia Medica with Repertory — Rs. 18.00

B. JAIN PUBLISHERS
Chronic Diseases and Theory of
Miasms — Rs. 4.50

BOSE, L.R.N. & KICHLU, K.L.
A Text Book of Descriptive Medicine
with Clinical Methods and
Homoeopathic Therapeutics — Rs. 25.00

CHOUDHARY, N.M.
A study on Materia Medica with
Repertory — Rs. 30.00

COWPERTHWEITE, A.C.
A Text Book of Gynaecology — Rs. 16.00
A Text Book of Materia Medica
and Therapeutics — Rs. 25.00

DEWEY, W.A.

GEORGE, ROYAL
Text Book of Homoeopathic Theory
and Practice of Medicine — Rs. 16.00

GROSS, H.
Comparative Materia Medica — Rs. 18.00

HAHNEMANN, SAMUEL
Organon of Medicine 6th Ed. — Rs. 7.20
Chronic Diseases (Theory) — Rs. 6.30

HERING, C.
The Homoeopathic Domestic Medicine — Rs. 9.50

HUGHES, R.
A Manual of Pharmacodynamics — Rs. 30.00

IYER, T.S.
Beginner's Guide to Homoeopathy — Rs. 15.00

JAHR, G.H.G.
Family Practice with Homoeopathic
Remedies — Rs. 6.50

KENT, J.T.
Repertory of the Homoeopathic
Materia Medica with Word Index — Rs. 32.50
Lectures on Homoeopathic Materia
Medica — Rs. 19.80
Lectures on Homoeopathic Philosophy — Rs. 8.10

LAURIE, J.
The Homoeopathic Practice of Medicine — Rs. 30.00
An Epitome of the Homoeopathic
Domestic Medicine — Rs. 15.00

MARSDON, J.H.
Hand-Book of Practical Midwifery — Rs. 11.00

MATHUR K.N.
Principles of Prescribing — Rs. 30.00

NASH, E.B.
Leaders in Homoeopathic Therapeutics — Rs. 8.50

ROBERT, H.